Skills *in*
Counselling &
Psychotherapy
with CHILDREN & YOUNG PEOPLE

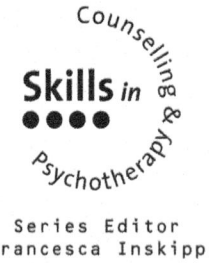

Series Editor
Francesca Inskipp

Skills in Counselling and Psychotherapy is a series of practical guides for trainees and practitioners. Each book takes one of the main approaches to therapeutic work or key client groups, and describes the relevant core skills and techniques.

Topics covered include:

- How to establish and develop the therapeutic relationship
- How to help the client change
- How to assess the suitability of an approach or technique for the client.

This is the first series of books to look at skills specific to the different theoretical approaches and is now developed to include skills specific to particular client groups. It is an ideal series for use on a range of courses which prepare the trainees to work directly with the clients.

Books in the series:

Skills in Cognitive Behaviour Therapy, Second Edition
Frank Wills

Skills in Gestalt Counselling and Psychotherapy, Third Edition
Phil Joyce and Charlotte Sills

Skills in Person-Centred Counselling and Psychotherapy, Second Edition
Janet Tolan

Skills in Psychodynamic Counselling and Psychotherapy
Susan Howard

Skills in Existential Counselling and Psychotherapy
Emmy van Deurzen and Martin Adams

Skills in Rational Emotive Behaviour Counselling and Psychotherapy
Windy Dryden

Skills in Transactional Analysis Counselling and Psychotherapy
Christine Lister-Ford

Skills in Solution Focused Brief Counselling and Psychotherapy
Paul Hanton

Skills *in* Counselling & Psychotherapy
with CHILDREN & YOUNG PEOPLE

Lorraine Sherman

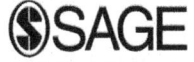

Los Angeles | London | New Delhi
Singapore | Washington DC

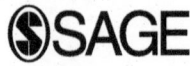

Los Angeles | London | New Delhi
Singapore | Washington DC

SAGE Publications Ltd
1 Oliver's Yard
55 City Road
London EC1Y 1SP

SAGE Publications Inc.
2455 Teller Road
Thousand Oaks, California 91320

SAGE Publications India Pvt Ltd
B 1/I 1 Mohan Cooperative Industrial Area
Mathura Road
New Delhi 110 044

SAGE Publications Asia-Pacific Pte Ltd
3 Church Street
#10-04 Samsung Hub
Singapore 049483

Editor: Kate Wharton
Assistant editor: Laura Walmsley
Production editor: Rachel Burrows
Marketing manager: Camille Richmond
Cover designer: Shaun Mercier
Typeset by: C&M Digitals (P) Ltd, Chennai, India
Printed in Great Britain by Henry Ling Limited at
The Dorset Press, Dorchester, DT1 1HD

© Lorraine Sherman 2015

First published 2015

Apart from any fair dealing for the purposes of research or private study, or criticism or review, as permitted under the Copyright, Designs and Patents Act, 1988, this publication may be reproduced, stored or transmitted in any form, or by any means, only with the prior permission in writing of the publishers, or in the case of reprographic reproduction, in accordance with the terms of licences issued by the Copyright Licensing Agency. Enquiries concerning reproduction outside those terms should be sent to the publishers.

Library of Congress Control Number: 2014938138

British Library Cataloguing in Publication data

A catalogue record for this book is available from the British Library

ISBN 978-1-4462-6016-6
ISBN 978-1-4462-6017-3 (pbk)

At SAGE we take sustainability seriously. Most of our products are printed in the UK using FSC papers and boards. When we print overseas we ensure sustainable papers are used as measured by the Egmont grading system. We undertake an annual audit to monitor our sustainability.

CONTENTS

About the Author	vii
Acknowledgements	viii
Introduction	1
Who is this book for?	1

1 Preparing for the Journey   5

Heart of practice – the therapeutic alliance	5
Basic competencies needed to begin	14
Liaising with adults	17
Theories into practice	19
Skills with different age groups	22

2 Assessing a Young Client   29

Dilemmas in assessment	29
Skills in completing assessment 'forms'	31
Assessing suitability for counselling	35
Including adults in referral processes	40

3 Deepening and Developing Counselling Skills   53

Skills in relating	54
Core elements of counselling skills	55
Developing the relationship	70

4 Extending Modalities to Counsel Children and Young People   81

Initial training	82
Integrative	83
Cognitive-behavioural	84
Psychodynamic	91
Person-centred and humanistic	95
Systemic	99
Narrative	100

5 Skills in Managing Professional Issues: Confidentiality and Disclosure, Agreements and Contracts   103

Confidentiality and disclosure	104
Explaining to parents/carers about confidentiality in counselling	107

	The legal framework	111
	Gillick competence	112
	Agreements and contracts	116
6	**Skills for Resolving Ethical Dilemmas**	**121**
	Applying the BACP Ethical Framework	122
	Understanding child protection	130
	School counsellors – independent or part of a pastoral team?	137
	Children and young people online – ethical practice and skills	138
7	**Skilful Play for Counsellors**	**143**
	Gaining confidence and ability with play	144
	The play journal	145
	Non-directed or directed play	148
	Different modalities' approach to play	148
	Adapting play methods to fit the circumstances of counselling	154
	Choosing play materials	157
	A counsellor's play kit	160
8	**Using Supervision Skilfully**	**165**
	Preparing for supervision	166
	One-to-one supervision – good practice do's and don'ts	170
	Group supervision	171
	The shape of supervision: Managerial, Educative and Restorative	173
	When we think we haven't acted well or have got it wrong	175
	Celebrating success	182
Index		184

ABOUT THE AUTHOR

Lorraine Sherman is a humanistic psychologist, supervisor, therapist, relationship counsellor and youth worker. She is clinical supervisor of school-based counsellors across West Wales. She has extensive experience in counselling and psychotherapeutic practice with young clients and adults. Lorraine designs and teaches courses to train counsellors and therapists to counsel children and young people. She lectures on counselling courses at Trinity St Davids University, Wales and has had many years of experience lecturing on the BACP accredited counselling courses based at Coleg Sir Gar, Ammanford. Lorraine includes mindfulness in her therapeutic work, she offers compassion-based approaches that include self-awareness, poetry and play and enjoys learning from her practice.

ACKNOWLEDGEMENTS

I wish to express my gratitude to:

Hazel Johns, my supervisor. Hazel encouraged me to write this book and believed I could do so throughout the process. Her ability to be consistently present, wise and helpful is astonishing. I am able to learn and grow through our supervisory relationship. I treasure meetings with her.

Francesca Inskipp, series editor, who has helped me get the reader's perspective, showing me how to communicate my ideas and make them accessible in written form. I feel fortunate to have received her insights as she read each chapter I wrote.

Shirley Sherman, my mum. Her clear accuracy when reading my writing meant she could find and correct spelling and grammatical errors. She perfectly balanced my passionate, intuitive style and helped me manage my undiagnosed dyslexic tendencies.

Colin Perrow, my husband and life companion, whose humour, kindness, love and unfailing support with everyday necessities have made writing this book a possibility for me. He has been powerfully encouraging through his belief in my work with children and young people. I couldn't have done it without him.

Jasmin Sherman-Perrow, my daughter, whose bright, theoretical mind and ability to express her emotions inspire me. Deep philosophical discussions with her in cafés have led me to re-examine some of my ideas about counselling children and young people. Her post-modern perspective is refreshing and insightful.

Kali, Nick, Ben, Tom and Layla Heaney, my Scottish family, who I play online games with, partly to research this book, but mostly for connection and fun. I am the Gran of their Clan!

My family in South East England, whom I have stayed with when meeting SAGE staff in Central London: my sister, Michele, with Stephen, James and Ricky in St Albans who welcome me, and my Dad in Muswell Hill who is a source of intelligent conversation.

Phil Layton and all at Area 43, Gill Dowsett and all at Theatr Fforwm Cymru, Simon O'Donohoe and all teaching colleagues, library staff and students at Coleg Sir Gar, thank you for good working relationships, friendship and opportunities to learn and grow in my therapeutic practice with children and young people.

Jules Heavens, mentor and ally, whose offer to help me get 'unstuck' with writing this book has enabled me to keep moving forward at difficult moments.

Kim Rosen, poetry teacher and facilitator, who has helped me get clear, enabling my writing to flow.

My peer supervisors, with whom I share my world of work and who restore and nourish me. Thanks particularly to Jenny Thompson and Pamela Gaunt for sharing their restorative homes with me.

••• Acknowledgements •••

All children and young people's counsellors and therapists whom I supervise, whose commitment to their counselling practice is extraordinary. I stand in awe of them. Two of those, Zena Cooper and Brigitte Osbourne, have contributed to the 'play kit' in this book.

Caroline Hepworth, Monique Kleinjans, Jane Bayley, Donna Williams, Alison Mott, Helena Blakemore, Samba Ndong and others, including the now departed Erin Macdonnell, for believing in me and helping me remember to smile.

Dene Donalds, mindfulness and meditation practice mentor, for his lightness, presence and sense of purpose.

The staff at SAGE, whose light, bright emails and welcoming words of encouragement have eased the journey.

Finally, heartfelt thanks to the memory of Peter Clarke (1948–2007), whose work as the First Children's Commissioner for Wales paved the way for a universal counselling service, entitling all children and young people aged 11–18 in Wales to access to a counsellor. He, with his team, advocated for independent, highly skilled, well trained counsellors based in all secondary schools in Wales. The Welsh Assembly put this into practice and the service exists today with so many children and young people benefitting. Peter's contribution is invisibly present on each page of this book.

INTRODUCTION

WHO IS THIS BOOK FOR?

This book is for counsellors, psychotherapists and others in helping professions who are in practice or aim to practise with children and young people. The contents have emerged out of many conversations and dialogues with others, including young people, in searching for the best way to counsel young clients.

A journey

Within the book is a journey you are invited to take:

- Meet a young client and begin a counselling relationship in Chapter 1.
- Consider how to assess and ensure clients are in the best place for them in Chapter 2.
- Examine counselling skills with children and young people in Chapter 3.
- Develop the particular modality you were trained in, so that you are able to counsel young clients skilfully, in Chapter 4.
- Discuss professional issues in Chapter 5, including the thorny issue of confidentiality with children and young people.
- Explore ethical dilemmas with young clients in Chapter 6.
- Discover skilful play in counselling in Chapter 7.
- Finally, make best use of supervision in Chapter 8.

A lifelong journey

For me, learning how to be with children and young people has been a lifelong journey. I have been a play leader, youth worker, college counsellor and a Relate counsellor before becoming a college lecturer in counselling and a supervisor. My time with Relate developed into being a trainer in the community, facilitating courses such as 'Parenting for Parents of Teenagers'. This allowed me to get a wider perspective on young people within their families.

My career with children and young people began as a 16-year-old play leader making up games in a hut in a London park. Aged 18, I began youth work and was fortunate enough to be taught communication skills from Transactional Analysis (TA) on a training day – skills I still use today.

Questioning assumptions

Members of the youth club where I worked showed me how to score at darts. I marvelled at how, although they were considered to be 'non-achievers' in school, they were so good at subtraction. Thus began my questioning of assumptions made about young people.

I worked in Tottenham on a play scheme. I met children who were called 'vandals' for piling up stones in a car park who would have been seen as having creative fun if there had been a river or beach for them to play the same games on. I shouted at people who were rude to 'our kids'. I was young and feisty, we played 'dirty word' scrabble, had serious water fights and painted with hands and bare feet on rolls of old wallpaper we had begged for from local shops.

Invisible baggage

I realised early on that lots of youngsters couldn't take advantage of opportunities offered to them because of invisible baggage they carried around. Beliefs that they were useless and worthless dogged their every step, often reinforced by adults around them. I knew about their glue sniffing and shop-lifting and the knives they carried. Taking knives away from fighting teenagers was normal then, though I would be more cautious now.

I didn't judge and I wasn't deluded into thinking they were angelic. We just got on, we fitted together. My early childhood had been a difficult one despite loving parents. At first shy and withdrawn and later angry and defiant, I became the street-wise rebellious teen that parents dread. When I played truant from school, I walked out of the front gate past the head's office and forged letters with my dad's signature. I didn't care what happened to me. I liked to be alone.

Despite the warning of my school's deputy head that I would fail my exams, I passed everything, luckily having a photographic memory that meant I could read one day, write it in an exam the next and then forget it all.

Eventually I ended up at university aged 22, and by this time I had met the ideas of Carl Rogers. I discovered a degree in 'Independent Studies' at Lancaster University and wrote my own syllabus called 'A Study of Human Potential'. A Philosophy tutor and a Politics tutor agreed to supervise my work. I studied Carl Rogers' writings at university in the early 1980s and I loved what I learnt.

Immediately after university, I qualified as a humanistic therapist; still in my twenties, I didn't practise as a therapist straightaway and continued my work with challenging young people.

••• Introduction •••

Discovering mindfulness

At this point I discovered mindfulness. A visiting tutor on my Humanistic Psychology diploma asked us what our daily practice was to replenish ourselves. No one reported a daily practice. I wanted one and needed to solve some problems left over from childhood. I studied and practised mindfulness then and I do so now. Mindfulness practice has sustained me for 30 years and is my teacher, central to my ability to continue being with young clients who have suffered abuse and neglect. I teach mindfulness to counsellors and am constantly learning and trying to live up to my own high standards! The book includes mindful moments, offering the opportunity to pause and refresh ourselves, whether we are reading or practising as counsellors and therapists.

Compassionate focus

Now, as a mature adult in my fifties, parent and grandparent, my aim is to be as responsible and compassionate in my everyday life as possible. I enjoy the change from being a rebellious risk taker but have not forgotten or suppressed the early experiences that formed me.

Twenty years ago, after moving to Wales with my partner and daughter, I began to counsel in a youth drop-in centre. This was the first time I had been given the opportunity to bring together my therapeutic skills and my experience with young people. I counselled courageous young people who had been abused and neglected, many of whom reported that they had not met anyone they could talk to or who would listen to them before.

Facilitating others

I was given the opportunity to develop and teach a Post-Qualifying Certificate in Counselling Young People. There is a session on the course where everyone becomes their inner adolescent and meets each other. It is not necessary to have had a misspent youth to complete this activity; to know the youth we once were is the aim!

Recently, whilst facilitating a supervision group, I offered to role-play my 10-year-old self so a counsellor could demonstrate a technique with emotional literacy cards. I arranged for one group member, a supervisor herself, to de-role me at the end of the exercise. I was amazed at how my 10-year-old self felt the urgency to speak to someone. I felt both the terror and relief of having someone to 'tell' and be with me non-judgementally.

The difference counselling makes for children and young people

My observer-self knew I had to monitor myself carefully in this exercise as I felt my inner 10-year-old's wish to disclose. During the role play, my 10-year-old self told the counsellor that there was 'something in one of the cards that she needed to talk about but couldn't say right now'. The counsellor kindly said, 'well, we will put that one aside and talk about it next time'. Relief swept over me. My 10-year-old self knew the opportunity to speak out was not lost.

As I de-roled, I realised the power of what had just happened and knew that I had experienced the difference that first contact with a skilled counsellor can make to children and young people.

Respect and the therapeutic alliance

It is the deep respect for and ability to join with children and young people that makes the difference. The therapeutic alliance is prioritised in this book, along with encouraging full comprehension of the legal and ethical aspects of counselling young clients in order for safe practice to take place.

Skills with different age groups are identified. The book covers counselling with children and young people starting at 5 years old and going on to 18. Stories of young clients in counselling moving through the different age groups of childhood and adolescence show us how to put the skills into practice.

The heart of practice

Helping children and young people through counselling is at the heart of this book. It is vital that the particular skills involved are recognised and practised.

There is no one kind of person that makes a good children and young people's counsellor. Whether your life experience is similar to mine or not, we will be able to come together and develop practice for the benefit of young clients.

The term 'counsellor' is used throughout to refer to the practitioner – it is hoped that psychotherapists and allied professionals will find the subject matter useful and recognise that, as the majority of readers will be counsellors, this is the preferable term to use.

Participative process

The reflective activities and mindful moments are designed for participation, either individually or in practitioner groups. Skills will be discovered through joining in and finding out what suits each of us and our particular circumstances in practice. Examples are based on experience and there is an invitation to engage with activities and processes used throughout the book.

1

PREPARING FOR THE JOURNEY

INTRODUCTION

In this chapter, we will consider what is needed to begin counselling children and young people. To be with a young person in the counselling room is both a privilege and a challenge – a privilege as there is the opportunity to know the intimate reality of a young human being's life and a challenge to make best use of the counselling and offer each young person the potential for growth and change.

At the heart of practice are the therapeutic processes and therapeutic alliance. On first meeting a young client, we need to consider how the therapeutic relationship is formed. What will be different in this relationship from being a parent, teacher or friend of the young person?

The creation of an alliance with young clients takes skill and practice.

HEART OF PRACTICE — THE THERAPEUTIC ALLIANCE

> ### CASE EXAMPLE: MAKING AN ALLIANCE WITH JAN
>
> Jan, aged 13, comes to your counselling room and begins by telling you she is 'fed up with do-gooders trying to help her'. How do you respond?

There are many possible responses to a statement like this one. What is the best approach to gain an alliance with Jan who has clearly had enough of the helping professions of which you are a member?

Three possible responses are:

1. 'Oh yeah, they are useless those social workers/teachers/mentors'. (child-to-child response) COLLUSION
2. 'Sounds like lots of people are trying to help you but you don't feel helped at all'. This response shows you have heard Jan and are giving her permission to express her dislike of what she perceives as 'do-gooders'.
3. 'Please don't speak like that here about people who want the best for you even if you are fed up with them'. (parent-to-child response) JUDGEMENT

Let us consider each of these responses in the light of establishing a therapeutic alliance. Would we feel tempted to offer the third or first response? What is wrong with doing so?

Response 1: here we are isolating ourselves from other professionals. When counselling children and young people, we may at times find ourselves blaming a teacher for shouting or a social worker for calling our client a 'drama queen'. It is easy to believe the client has a right to have an adult on 'their side' and this validates statement 1. If you believe an adult is acting in an inappropriate way towards your young client, it is vital to act. This needs to be done with calm and clear empathetic responses and not by joining in with a client's anger or rejection of authority.

Response 3: challenging young people who behave in rude and sullen ways invites 'critical parent' responses. If we do respond in this way, it is probably the last time we will see Jan, having been written off by her as someone trying to reform her behaviour, rather than get to know her empathically.

Response 2: we need to get alongside Jan, finding in us the place where we can really connect with what it is like to be her. This is what the second response begins to do.

What comes next? Jan is still eyeing us with suspicion, waiting to be told off or for you to attempt to help her. How do you build the therapeutic alliance from this place?

A useful strategy is to stick to honest and clear facts, for the first few minutes, about the possibilities and limitations available in counselling. This helps to deal with the 'bullshit detector' that young people often have in abundance. Honesty includes explaining the counselling contract to Jan at this early stage. This is part of being empathic in that it shows the client you know what it is like to BE them. Jan will probably appreciate clarity and honesty, both of which are often in short supply in a young person's life.

Emotional literacy

We have the potential to open a door to a whole new world for a young person. The 'norms' of the counselling room may be very distant from a young client's everyday life. Emotional literacy is still not very widespread. You may find that a minority of your clients are exceptionally well versed in the language of feelings. A child or young person who has grown up in a home that allows and encourages expressions of anger, sadness, happiness and joy will have developed emotional literacy. A young client who is emotionally literate can say, for example, if they feel envious of a sibling or sad at the death of a pet. More often, there has been selective permission to feel some feelings and not others. Sadness is acceptable, but anger is not or anger is expressed so unskilfully as to be linked to aggression. Sometimes substances are used in families as ways to suppress feelings, and these may be legal or illegal.

Some children and young people will have already learnt in their early years that the expression of how they feel about anything puts them in danger of punishment. These young people have become able to hide how they really feel and sometimes will have lost connection with what it means to genuinely express emotion. A safe survival response to the circumstances in which they have grown up could be to hide feelings, manipulate situations or close down emotional responses. Young clients may have learnt to try to give adults what they think is wanted by them rather than express their real needs or wants. Conversely, they may have decided that any attention is better than none and act in odd or defiant ways to be noticed.

Suddenly, as the young client enters the counselling room for the first time, they enter a place where feelings have value, openness is encouraged and privacy respected. The newness and difference from everyday life should not be under-estimated.

Skills and qualities

There are various skills and qualities that the young people's counsellor needs to bring to a first session to establish a relationship. An acronym for these is: H. E. A. R. O. S.:

Holding the Overview

Empathy

Age-appropriateness

Resilience

Openness to Difference

Self-care

Some of these skills will be familiar ones to all counsellors. They need to be practised in a new manner within the context of counselling children and young people.

Considering each in turn with examples can help to clarify and illuminate how to use these skills.

Holding the overview

This is an area that illustrates that counselling with children and young people is clearly different from counselling adults. When we counsel adults, we allow them to make choices concerning who they live with and how they conduct their personal relationships. A young person has far less choice in these matters, often none at all.

Reluctance, nervousness and ambivalence about attending counselling can all be managed and often overcome. Ongoing coercion, threats or bribes to attend, however, are not a good basis for creating a therapeutic alliance.

During the first session:

- Establish the nature of counselling with the young client.

- Let new clients know that you are not going to try to 'make' them behave differently.

- Be prepared to listen, find out what it is like to be the young client and enable them to understand their situation and life choices.

- Be yourself – this is vital in these initial stages as is an open account of the limitations of the service you are offering.

- Explain clearly the limits to confidentiality and the time constraints. This is considered in detail later in this book (in Chapter 5).

- Ask your client if they have had counselling or therapy before.

- Offer a different approach – sometimes young people are referred to see professionals and they have very little idea about who that professional is and what is going to happen.

- Take the time to explain who you are and what it is you hope for in the counselling process.

- Offer a general explanation of what you will and will not be doing in counselling.

- Include the opportunity for young clients to ask any questions they would like to.

Remember that it may be the first time in the young person's life that they have had one-to-one time with an adult they do not know. Once trust is established, this can be a great opportunity, though initially it may seem strange. The environment in which you meet your young client needs to aid this first contact.

REFLECTIVE ACTIVITY: FINDING THE OVERVIEW

Remember a time in your childhood or youth when you held a differing view to your parents or teachers but were made to do what they told you to.

Can you recall how you *felt*? Note the feelings down.

Now as an adult, how do you perceive that same situation looking back?

If the two views differ, attempt to see both views simultaneously, as if from a third position, as a neutral observer. Hold a sense of valuing everyone in the situation.

This is the overview – a place of compassion and care for each person involved.

Empathy

The skill of being empathic with a young person is particularly important. We need to step into their world and gain comprehension of what it is like to be their age in their particular circumstances. Our own expectations and beliefs will be barriers to this, however open we are.

Being in the present with your young client is a good way to begin the empathic connection that you need to find in order to build the therapeutic alliance.

Child 'ego state' The transactional analysis child 'ego state' is helpful in understanding how to do this (Stewart and Joines 2012). The child ego state is divided into 'free' and 'adapted' child. One useful aspect of TA is the explicit explanation of words, gestures and postures that identify the child state. A child-to-child transaction will help us to connect with the young client, though as young person's therapists we need to be vigilant that we don't over-identify and remain clearly as the counsellor or therapist, not trying to be friend, playmate or 'partner in crime'!

Empathising with the young client involves allowing our own inner child to be present whilst always remembering we are no longer a child.

Age-appropriateness

The age of the client will give many clues as to how to respond to them. The language used with a 6-year-old will be different to the language employed with a 16-year-old. Later in the chapter, counselling different age groups will be examined in depth. Age appropriate language and responses by young people's counsellors are an important aspect of the counselling.

A family divorce is a good example of this:

> A young child aged between 5 and 9 years, needs to know that there will be continued security for them. Young children might believe that they have done something to upset their parents, feeling they have caused the divorce by not putting toys away, for example. The counsellor needs to respond appropriately, perhaps saying 'mummy and 'daddy' when speaking of the parents if this is what the child calls them.

> A 10–13-year-old may be more angry and confused concerning the divorce; they won't want their friendship groups disturbed if they need to move house. The counsellor needs to accept the emerging adolescent's frustrations, adapting to the client's use of language.

> A 14–18-year-old often blames parents and finds fault with them during a divorce. Some of this age group want to move out, stay with friends or protect younger siblings. The counsellor notices adulthood emerging in the client and offers an alliance whilst parents are occupied in separating.

It may seem self-evident that different responses are required, but young children in particular are often burdened by being given adult choices about which parent they want to live with or with tales of who did what to whom. There are some age-appropriate choices that are good; too much choice can be terrifying.

Resilience

Resilience is a skill that involves staying flexible and emotionally balanced. It may seem as if counselling and therapy work with children and young people is an easy option, but this is far from the truth. It can bring a counsellor into contact with their own feelings of loss and pain when young clients are suffering deeply. Of course, this is balanced by the fun and lightness of childhood and youth. Playing games, laughing and making jokes are part of counselling children and young people as well.

Often, we cannot change a child's life circumstances that seem from our intimate knowledge of them to be woefully inadequate.

CASE EXAMPLE: SUSIE AT RISK

Susie is 12 and living with her step-father; her mother has left and is not in contact with the family. Susie disclosed some months ago that her step-father was touching her inappropriately. Her step-father was arrested but the case was dropped and social services decided Susie should remain at home. Susie tells you that her step-grandmother is furious with her and told her she will not be having presents at Christmas because of what she said about her step-father. Susie is frightened and upset. She makes it clear to you that her step-father did behave in an abusive manner toward her.

This type of case raises concerns for us. We can follow procedures and make child protection referrals but usually we are not able to act alone to protect the young client and rely on other professionals' assessment of any particular situation. Though there can be re-referrals and a counsellor should continue to offer the child's perspective once a disclosure has been made, sometimes the child remains in a situation that seems inappropriate from the counsellor's perspective (see Chapter 5 on disclosure).

Counselling children makes us particularly prone to feeling the need to 'take charge' and act on behalf of the child or young person. It is exceptionally easy to find oneself in the position of protector, advocate, advisor, parent or educator. Counsellors often want to change children or young people's lives. The counsellor may find that active roles are included in practice with young people. The principle of beneficence in the BACP Ethical Framework enables recognition of the circumstances when there is a need to act 'in the best interests' of the client. This aspect of counselling is explored in depth in Chapters 5 and 6. Actions taken can be complex and take time and energy to resolve. This requires the counsellor to be stable and remain calm in challenging circumstances.

Sometimes counsellors keep confidentiality because a teenage client wishes a matter to be kept private. The counsellor may think the client could receive help if they were willing to disclose, but if there are no child protection concerns then the client's wishes can be respected.

Counsellors of children or young people face witnessing their difficult and challenging life. This requires skills in resilience:

- Notice how you are affected and influenced by the young client's issues.
- Gain appropriate support if a child or young person's story has disturbed you.
- Recognise that you may become distressed because of a sense of being unable to change the external circumstances of the client.
- When the counselling relationship is becoming established and rapport develops, you may want to change the child or young person's life. This change may not be possible and managing difficult circumstances with the young client requires resilience.

Key methods of support to gain resilience include supervision, personal counselling or therapy and strategies to prevent 'burn-out'.

Supervision The subject of supervision is fully discussed in Chapter 8. In the context of establishing a relationship with your client, it is necessary to check that your supervisor is well versed in young people's issues and has had therapeutic experience in counselling and/or therapy with under 18s.

Personal counselling or therapy Issues raised when counselling young people may bring to the fore a need for therapeutic support. Where the young client has similar circumstances to those from the counsellor's early life and these are unresolved, there is often a need to address this therapeutically.

Strategies for prevention of 'burn-out' Symptoms of 'burn-out', such as feeling exhausted, overwhelmed and unable to cope, should be recognised early. Treat these as useful warning signs. Talk to others, do not try to struggle on alone and remember that it is not uncommon to feel like this when counselling young clients. It is good to pay attention to the reality that the young client may have come from a very disturbed home environment and that this atmosphere will have an effect on you. Rothschild (2006) gives us the concept of 'mirror neurons' as a way of explaining vicarious traumatisation. This means that bodies pick up the difficult feelings of others and counsellors can be left disturbed and upset long after a client has left. Weiss (1999) offers personal and professional strategies for 'burn-out prevention'. These include:

- playing when we are not at work
- having emotionally supportive people around us who are thinking about other things besides therapy
- having an early warning system for our own emotional state
- attending to physical health, exercise, good food and sleep.

Openness to difference

The skill of being 'open to difference' means raising our awareness of assumptions made about children and young people. Most young people's counsellors are advocates *for* young people and hold positive views about their clients. This alone does not prevent counsellors from making assumptions about a particular client outside of conscious awareness. We can usefully question beliefs, opinions and ideas about children and young people. When a young client enters the counselling room, we may make decisions about them very quickly based on their clothing, eye contact or lack of it, their smell or the manner in which they enter the room. These assumptions are part of being human and based on life experience and self-protection.

Assumptions A friend was nervous travelling home in the evening because of young people with brightly coloured hair on public transport. When I said to her that I knew young people who were shy, quiet and studious with hair dyed extraordinary bright colours, she was very surprised!

Make notes of the kinds of assumptions you might make or have made concerning children and young people.

Is a 7-year-old girl with long blonde hair 'sweet'? Possibly, but there needs to be an openness in counsellors to question themselves so as not to stereotype and assume according to beliefs. The skill of being open to the world view of the young enables the client to reveal who they are, without being judged or being subjected to assumptions. Take the example of an A-grade student who is self-harming. A counsellor brings this client to supervision, saying they are surprised because 'he's so bright, he's not the type to self-harm'. This shows assumptions and a lack of openness to who this client actually is.

Adolescents particularly suffer from being 'pigeon-holed' because of their appearance. The openness of the counsellor and a willingness to wait and see who the client is, is a useful skill that takes practice. The nature of our young client group means there may be many differences between counsellor and client. These include:

- age
- values
- culture
- beliefs
- attitudes
- priorities
- communication style.

This wide divergence, explored throughout the book, means there is a need to develop a variety of new skills and offer personal qualities in order to develop a therapeutic alliance.

Self-care

Self-care involves taking care of our own 'issues' as counsellors. When preparing for the counselling journey, consider:

- Is your client the same age as one of your children?
- Is your client bringing an issue that affected you in your own childhood?
- Are you able to counsel this particular young client?
- Are you gaining the support you need?

When counselling young clients, self-care can be enhanced through being mindful.

Mindfulness is 'The awareness that emerges through paying attention, on purpose and non-judgementally, to the unfolding of experience moment to moment' (Kabat Zinn 2003: 145). Being mindful offers the opportunity to fully recognise our part in the counselling relationship, noticing our own reactions and being both reflective and responsible for our actions.

A mindful counsellor is able to exercise self-care and take appropriate breaks between clients. Counsellors sometimes take a short walk or a few moments of quiet space to breathe. These activities help to clear the mind and bring us the clarity and freshness needed to welcome the next client.

> **MINDFUL MOMENT: SELF-CARE EXERCISE — THE 'BREATHING SPACE'**
>
> Sit in an upright, comfortable position. Notice the rise and fall of your breath. Bring yourself into the here and now, letting go of thoughts of the previous client and relaxing your body as best you can. If your mind is carried into thoughts of the past or the future, just notice this and bring yourself once again into the present. After a few minutes, continue with your next activity.

This exercise is for the counsellor's benefit, just to practise alone to prepare for the next part of the day. It is not recommended that counsellors offer mindfulness exercises to clients unless they have a well-established mindfulness practice in their everyday life.

Being fully present with a young client is an aspect of self-care that can be brought to counselling. Self-care can be a way of caring for our client too. If we are in good spirits, refreshed and ready for each young person who comes into the counselling room, then we are honouring our commitment to the counselling process. This requires counsellors to 'sharpen' their own awareness and recognise the lack of selfishness in prevention of burn-out.

Mindful presence is considered further in Chapter 3, where the developing and deepening of the counselling relationship are explored.

BASIC COMPETENCIES NEEDED TO BEGIN

There are basic principles and requirements that need to be in place for the safe grounds of a skilful alliance between counsellor and young client to develop. Skills and knowledge are needed before starting to counsel children and young people. These include:

◆ suitable qualifications and experience
◆ knowledge of relevant laws, rights of the child and referral procedures.

Qualifications

Practically, it is necessary for counsellors working with young clients to be fit for purpose. Specific training and qualifications are essential. The initial, generic training that most counsellors and therapists receive is aimed at working with adults. This type of training on its own is not sufficient for counselling children and young people. Chapter 4 is dedicated to exploring how to extend an initial counselling qualification to counselling children and young people. We need to recognise at the outset that, as counsellors, we are not fully prepared to counsel younger clients unless we have trained to do so.

Experience

Knowing how to relate to young clients comes from experience both inside and outside the counselling room. We were all young once and remembering clearly what it was like to be a child and then a teenager is an asset. Sometimes the memory of being young is overridden by a critical or nurturing parental attitude or by adult, rational processes that block out memories of childhood and adolescence.

REFLECTIVE ACTIVITY: WHAT ARE OUR OPINIONS?

Complete the phrases:
 'Children are............' and 'Young people are................' for yourself and then ask the same of others you know.
  Change the phrase to: 'Teenagers are...........'.
  Then respond to:
 'Girls are............' and 'Boys are...............'.
  Try not to censor the initial answers, as they give such interesting information, even though we may not always approve of our own beliefs and may want to modify any

biases. In this way, life experiences and knowledge of what we believe can be brought into awareness.

A sense of 'society's views' of children and young people is also useful for counsellors to have.

Being a parent or teacher or having counselled adults is insufficient experience alone to counsel children and young people. Youngsters need counsellors with plenty of relevant training, skills and experience. Counselling the young is far from easy and there are responsibilities that need skilful application.

Children and young people, in many cases, cannot and do not pay for their own counselling and counselling for this age group can sometimes be undertaken with low paid or voluntary counsellors. Whilst many of these counsellors will have plenty of excellent experience and ability, it is vital to recognise, across the profession, that specialised training is needed when counselling this potentially vulnerable client group.

Law

It is vital to understand the law as it currently applies to minors in counselling and how the particular environment of the counselling, such as a school, youth club or private practice, will change what is required of us. This aspect of counselling children and young people will be explained in depth in Chapter 5 which looks at confidentiality, disclosure and sharing concerns. It is necessary to be aware of the relevant law before we enter the counselling room with a young person for the first time. Finding it out later is not an acceptable option! If a young client is at risk of significant harm, the correct procedure needs to be followed and that client needs to know how any actions taken by the counsellor will affect them.

Rights

Young people have rights, but they are able to say what they do and do not want in their lives only to a limited extent. Young people are often subject to the rules and decisions of adults. This creates a marked difference between those counselling adults and those young people. There is an inevitable inequality in the counselling relationship that needs to be skilfully addressed by the child and young person's counsellor.

Referral procedures

Counselling is a voluntary activity, yet the young person coming for the first time may not be able to choose their appointment time or place. The appointment might be when their parent can bring them or when the school will release them from class. The decision about their attendance may have been made by an adult. Some young people do self-refer; however, it is useful to take into account that it is unlikely that many of your young clients will have chosen to come in the way that adult clients do. What does this mean as a counsellor of a child or young person? Instantly, it can be recognised that there are differences in making a therapeutic alliance with young people when compared to making an alliance with adult clients.

Ensuring counselling is voluntary

We need to consider whether a young client has been given options about attending counselling or not. How do we ensure there is agreement by the child or young person themselves? The answer to this may seem simple: we ask clients and they choose whether to come to counselling or not. In fact, ways that young clients get to counselling vary enormously and some have no idea what counselling is or even that you are a counsellor when they attend their first appointment. Introducing what counselling is requires skill, and explaining that clients have a choice about attending is necessary. Children and young people need information to ascertain whether this unknown activity, called 'counselling', is worthwhile.

Access to counselling

Many schools in Britain and all secondary schools in Wales have a counsellor available to pupils. Children's rights legislation, including the 1989 Children's Act, has enabled a new and different understanding of the right of a child to receive confidential counselling. Case law has consistently upheld the principle that young people who are mature enough to give informed consent can receive counselling without permission being given by an adult. Young people can and do refer themselves to counselling, both in schools and in youth clubs and drop-in centres.

REFLECTIVE ACTIVITY: EARLIEST KNOWLEDGE OF COUNSELLING

When did you first know about counselling? What age were you? How did you think and feel about counselling then?

Just allow your first answers to come to mind; if you are not sure, just imagine how you might have thought or felt about counselling.

Imagine yourself as a child going to counselling: What might you have spoken about to your counsellor? Get a sense of what counselling would have meant to you as a child.

Note down your responses and share them, if you wish, with a trusted colleague or your supervisor.

LIAISING WITH ADULTS

We need to learn skills in liaising with the adults responsible for our young clients. More information about this is found throughout the book. In the initial stages of meeting your young client:

- Listen to the concerns of those who wish the child or young person to have counselling. You may need to speak with the adult responsible for enabling the young client to attend. There may be financial, transport or collection issues.

- Speak to the referring adult separately to make necessary practical arrangements. NEVER speak 'over the head' of a child or young person as if they were not there.

> ### CASE EXAMPLE: THE YOUNG CLIENT IN PRIVATE PRACTICE
>
> The mother of a 12-year-old boy, Liam, phones to ask if you can counsel her son. She describes the boy as being 'very angry'.
> How do you form a relationship with this boy when your first contact is with his mother, the person with whom he is currently having a very challenging relationship?

We need to cultivate the skill of diplomacy to make a therapeutic alliance with Liam whilst also communicating openly with his mother when necessary.

To create the environment necessary for a parent or carer to trust a counsellor with their child, mutual respect is vital. Taking sides – either by joining with the referring adult and believing 'stories' about behaviour and 'problems' in the client or by siding with the young client in criticising their parents – can be detrimental to forming a therapeutic relationship. If an adult is behaving in an abusive manner, then a different response is necessary (see Chapter 5 on confidentiality).

Recent research on schools-based counselling has shown that whether the young client chooses counselling or is referred, the outcomes can be positive. The research shows that it is not absolutely necessary for Liam to be 'on board' at this stage. Counselling is voluntary; an educated choice involves him knowing what and who he is choosing. If after the first session Liam expresses a clear wish not to attend again, then this needs to be respected. At this point, though, some reticence and questioning of the counselling are to be expected and understood.

On hearing a young client's story, we must be careful to recognise that what they are saying is true in their experience. Our own age and experience may give us a different view of the issue. You might be a parent yourself and have been through similar issues with your own children. A teenager not allowed out after 11pm may consider their parent to be cruel. A teenager regularly being beaten and punched by their parent may feel that they deserve this treatment and forgive the parent. This kind of dilemma can rise up instantly and very early on in the therapeutic relationship. Here, the counsellor needs to hold the overview by not agreeing with the client that abuse is acceptable; conversely there may be a need to challenge the view the client holds that having boundaries about reasonable times to be home is cruel.

Sometimes we must consider our own values, those of our profession and how the law protects children during the first few moments of meeting our client.

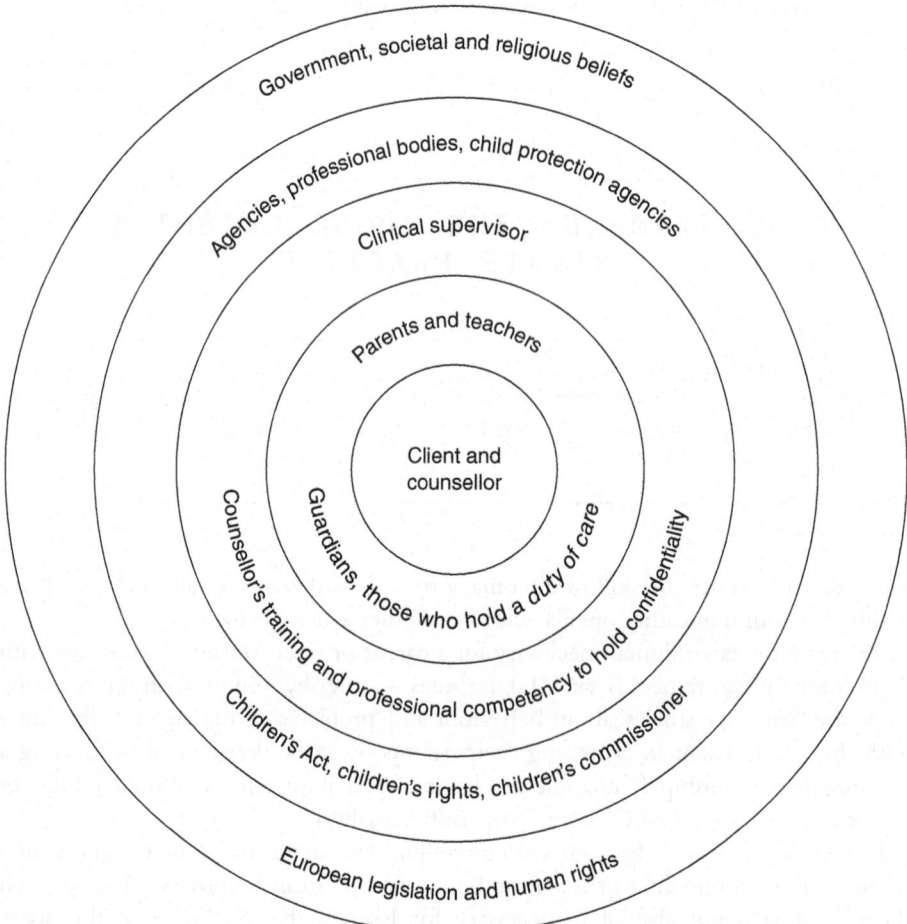

Figure 1   Who is in the room?

All these layers are present, though invisible, when the counsellor forms a therapeutic relationship with a young client. It is necessary to highlight them in order to consider how the client being young, a minor in law, changes the manner in which the forming of a relationship takes place. Confidentiality can be maintained in most cases with an older child who is competent to consent (see Chapter 5). There may, however, be a requirement to share more information concerning a young child. This particular skill requires the counsellor to hold at least two perspectives at any one time. Valuing the young person's feelings and experience whilst recognising other, often competing views of the situation takes great skill (see Chapter 6).

THEORIES INTO PRACTICE

Geldard and Geldard (2010) give a useful overview of theories beginning with Maslow's Hierarchy of Needs. In this chapter, how these theories are applied is shown through case examples. Many counsellors will be familiar with Maslow from early on in their training as a counsellor. This theory is not specific to children and young people but can usefully be applied to the young. Maslow identified a pyramid and gives us insight into an order in which the process of self-actualisation can occur. Basic needs for food, shelter and belonging must be present before a child or young person can begin the journey of self-discovery.

Maslow

> **CASE EXAMPLE: RECOGNISING A CLIENT'S 'HIERARCHY OF NEEDS'**
>
> Clare is referred to you in a youth drop-in centre. She is 16 and is 'sofa surfing', staying with friends as her family situation has become too difficult for her to remain at home. This is her first session with you and as her story unfolds it becomes clear that she has not eaten a meal other than snacks in the last 24 hours. She then confides to you that she has her period but has no money to buy sanitary protection and is trying to manage by using loo roll.

To establish a counselling relationship with Clare:

- encourage her to talk to the youth workers about her current situation
- ask her for her agreement so you can talk to relevant agencies who will offer her help with her basic needs
- ensure she knows you will be there to counsel her although there are practical concerns
- use straightforward language to explain things – for example, just say: 'as you are really hungry that's the first thing to sort out; when you are more comfortable we can talk some more'.

Applying Maslow's hierarchy is helpful here as it is evident that Clare's needs for food, shelter and sanitary protection should be addressed before the counselling can progress.

Erikson

The 'life stage' theory of Erik Erikson (1995) helps in counselling children as we can gain a sense of how a young person's struggle to gain independence can be a useful resolution of a developmental crisis which is in fact part of 'growing up' to the next stage of life. Erikson gave us the term 'identity crisis' for adolescents. His contribution has enabled an understanding of the young person trying to find out who they are, as opposed to who they are told to be by adults, and viewing this as a positive process rather one to be feared.

> **CASE EXAMPLE: IDENTITY CRISIS**
>
> Jon comes to see you; he is studying for his A levels at college and is enjoying the uniform-free environment. He is in his third term now and has found a new group of friends, who all wear black. Jon is dressed totally in black and has black nail varnish on a couple of his fingers. He has his hood up when he comes into the counselling room, looks at the floor a lot and tells you that his mum is 'freaking out' and telling him he is going to 'waste his life' and 'come to nothing'. Jon doesn't want to upset his mum but there is 'no way' he is going to give up his new friends.

For Jon, it is the aim of his developmental stage to resolve role confusion and find himself. Erikson tells us that time and space are needed for Jon to develop. Jon's new views bring him into conflict with his mum and in counselling he can express himself and find a way to maintain a relationship with his mother. The therapeutic alliance, starting the counselling journey with Jon, is best served by being alongside him in his journey to find his identity without either colluding with him 'against' his mum or trying to make him change to placate her. This role can be so important to the developing adolescent who then feels understood.

Piaget and Kohlberg

As counsellors of children, we need to understand that they gain skills at particular ages. Piaget (2001) observed children and noticed distinct differences in what they can conceptualise depending on their age. Asking a child under 11 to consider something in abstract terms is inappropriate as it will be beyond their ability. As a counsellor beginning a relationship with a child of 9 or 10, it is necessary to accept that though the ability to understand another's view has developed, the capacity to make decisions about their own future will be beyond their developmental stage. There are additional stages of moral development, outlined by Kohlberg (1984): these start at stage one – avoiding punishment – and go through to stages involving mutual respect and universal, ethical principles.

When forming relationships with children, the counsellor's skills will be enhanced by understanding the child's developmental stage. A young client aged 10, for example,

Bowlby's attachment theory

The current widely held belief that a young child needs consistent contact with a primary caregiver, usually the mother, is based on Bowlby's attachment theory. Hospital beds are often provided for parents to stay when their children are admitted. Usually there is plenty of visiting time and a commonly held belief that this contact with the primary person with whom the child has bonded is very important. It is also true that before the theory of attachment was well known and accepted, it was generally thought that a nurse could offer the full care needed by a young child in hospital and visiting by parents was restricted (Bowlby 1988; see also Chapter 4 on extending the counselling modality you were trained in).

Other cultures emphasise extended family care and parents are sometimes less involved than grandparents. Bowlby's theory may be limited in value in counselling these clients, as secure attachment may come from belonging to an extended family or village culture.

CASE EXAMPLE: ATTACHMENT ISSUES

Natalie, aged 6, has been sent to see you because she is very nervous and withdrawn at school. After a year of being in school, she still cries a lot when her mum leaves her. She finds it hard to make friends. You are given the information that Natalie's mum has suffered with cancer for the past four years and has been hospitalised a number of times. Natalie has been 'well cared for' by a variety of friends and family during her mum's time as an inpatient in hospital.

In a case such as this, allow the child to:

- just play and explore the counselling environment
- form a relationship with you
- find security in the structure of and lack of demands on her in counselling.

Natalie does not have to talk about or understand the loss she has probably felt due to her mum's absence. The process of play and being with the counsellor is a vital part of the counselling in this case.

SKILLS WITH DIFFERENT AGE GROUPS

The following are some skills in preparing for the counselling journey with children and young people of different ages:

can be 'rule bound', wanting to get everything right and full of feelings that everything is 'not fair', so the counsellor may want to encourage the client to question these attitudes. It is useful to consider that this may be the 'conventional' moral stage of development outlined by Kohlberg (1984).

> **George** is 10, he has two younger siblings and both he and his parents want him to have an opportunity to learn computer skills and he now has a laptop. George's parents are worried by what he might see if he goes on the internet. George doesn't know what his parents are worried about, as he just wants to play a few games and link up with friends in an online building game. George's parents turn off the internet in the house and refuse to give him the password or discuss the matter with him. He is only allowed online when a parent is by his side. George has secretly learnt the password and sneaks time on the internet. In counselling, he is concerned because his parents don't trust him and he thinks of himself as a 'good' boy; he is confused and doesn't like his own sneaky behaviour.

Here, it can be seen that the cognitive and moral development stages are relevant to considering how to manage this case. The client's own view of right and wrong and that he would not do anything deliberately 'bad' brings him into a difficult moral dilemma. Does he sneak or forfeit his time online? As counsellors, we can see that his parents' refusal to talk with him about the concerns they have for his safety online is a factor in a difficult situation for George. It is often true that parents and those responsible for children's wellbeing don't want them to 'grow up too quickly' and explaining what the dangers might be for George would potentially involve a conversation about sex, pornography and grooming. Unintended consequences, the aspects of the situation that George does not yet understand, influence the decisions of the adults around him, including the counsellor.

An ethical dilemma then arises for the counsellor. Is George 'at risk' on the internet in this way? As he is probably too young to make such decisions, do his parents need to know straightaway? It can be seen here that a moral dilemma in the child can lead to a similar dilemma for the counsellor.

The counsellor may want to encourage George to ask his parents why using the internet alone is forbidden. The suggestion of a meeting with the parents and George so he can ask his question with the counsellor present may also be possible in some contexts.

Telling George in very simple terms that not everyone is kind to children and he must not be in contact online with anyone who he doesn't know is useful but may not be enough. There is a cause for concern here that requires the counsellor to consider all the issues and whether confidentiality must be broken. This dilemma is closely connected with George's age, on the 'cusp' between childhood and early adolescence.

Skills to apply:

◆ Accept the client's stage of development whilst keeping an awareness of their individuality.

◆ Be present as the counsellor whilst holding an awareness of the 'child protector' role.

5 to 9 years

Young children will expect their counsellor to be an adult who is in charge. Children may initially be surprised that you are offering time, space, attention and attentive listening, as well as a place to play and 'be' rather than 'do'. Skills with this age group include:

- softened eye contact, smiling and reassuring
- physically being on the child's level, sitting on a low chair or on cushions
- explaining who you are and what counsellors do
- letting the child know what the limits and 'rules' of the counselling room are, e.g. how long each week they will be with you, who will collect them from you, what you will be sharing with their parent/carer or teacher and what is just between the two of you.

10 to 13 years

Skills with this age group include:

- responding to the early adolescent, managing embarrassment due to new levels of 'self-consciousness' and the need for privacy
- transition issues, new school, child towards adulthood, the loss of childhood, bodily changes, the importance of peer group and new disagreements with parents/teachers, those in authority
- allowing the young person to be 'expert' on their experience whilst holding a recognition of the possible 'unintended consequences' of their choices
- letting the young person know you are worthy of respect through clear boundaries in the counselling room.

14 to 18 years

Skills with this age group include:

- getting alongside the client, forming a therapeutic alliance
- recognising the adolescent need for independence, more sleep, exploring sexuality and the responsibilities of adult life
- explicitly talking with the client about their emerging adulthood, responsibilities, exams, money, planned career, training or university
- showing respect for the client's difficulties, using plenty of empathy
- never belittling dilemmas even if the attitudes seem odd or extreme

- offering a different approach to other adults, challenging where necessary whilst respecting that the client knows and understands their own situation

- allowing yourself to enter the 'teenage' world, see through their eyes and feel how it is to be in their position before offering any interventions or solutions

- encouraging the emerging adult by creating an equal relationship as a 'model' for how the client can approach people or situations in their life.

Skills in responding to children as unique individuals

Responses to individual children and young people vary; one 12-year-old, for example, can be very much a child, physically and emotionally, whilst another can be well advanced into puberty, at their full adult height and experiencing hormonal changes that influence their emotional responses. Gender and circumstantial differences need to be taken account of. A traumatised child may display behaviours relating to a different age group than would be expected of their chronological years. The skills offered above relating to age groups are guidelines that should be applied intelligently and flexibly. It is the counsellor's responsibility not to expect too much from a young child or respond in a belittling manner to a young person.

CASE EXAMPLE: TRAUMA

Angela, aged 10, is brought to the counselling room by the school 'link' person. As soon as the counselling room door is closed, Angela flattens herself against the door, wide-eyed and silent. Suggestions made that she might like to sit down are ignored and, after a few minutes, Angela begins to roam around the room, picking up objects and occasionally making sounds.

In a case like this, it becomes clear that the counsellor needs to respond to what is happening in the counselling room and not use any understanding based on the chronological age of the client.

Angela is showing signs and symptoms of trauma and this requires the counsellor to offer a calm presence and the ability to allow what may seem to be 'odd' or 'disturbed' behaviours to unfold without rushing the child.

Levine (2010) offers five principles to guide children's play toward resolution of trauma. The principles are:

1. Let the child control the pace of the game.

2. Distinguish between fear, terror and excitement.

3. Take one small step at a time.
4. Become a safe container.
5. Stop if you feel the child is genuinely not benefiting from the play.

These principles can be applied to counselling traumatised children. In the case of Angela, the principles are useful in enabling the counsellor to respond in a skilful and appropriate manner.

1 Let the child control the pace of the game

Angela eventually settles on play dough and begins to make biscuits and birthday cakes. She still speaks very little and is not making much eye contact with you. What she does say are repetitions of words from a video shown to the whole school in assembly that morning.

2 Distinguish between fear, terror and excitement

Angela is frightened; it seems her terror which was present when she first entered the room is subsiding.

> If the child appears frightened or cowed, give reassurance but don't encourage any further movement. Instead, be present with your full attention and support, waiting patiently until a substantial amount of the fear subsides. (Levine 2010: 208)

Some of Angela's behaviour could be misinterpreted as 'naughty'. One example of this is her turning the light on and off in the counselling room. It is necessary to make sure Angela remains safe throughout her activities whilst recognising she is trying to resolve her fears and traumatic memories.

3 Take one small step at a time

As the session with Angela develops, it is clear she is starting to relax and enjoy the play. She becomes very involved and does not want to stop at the end of her counselling time. Gradually and slowly, we are able to draw the session to a close.

On returning Angela to her classroom, other professionals express surprise and compliment you that she has engaged in the counselling process in any way, commenting on the length of time she was with you, her usually short attention span and often blunt refusal to communicate with helping professionals.

A request is made that you try to find out what her 'wishes are' as she is a 'looked after' child in foster care at present. Whilst this request is made in good faith, it is far too early to ask any questions of this type of Angela in counselling. Crossing Angela's boundaries and trying to make her talk about her 'wishes' would comply with 'norms' of managing Angela's 'case'. It would be inappropriate and ineffective to push her into this and counter-productive as she has clearly learnt how to defend herself when she doesn't want to talk or feels it would be dangerous to do so. Much of the way Angela reacts is not within her conscious control; rather it is an instinctual response to the difficulties she has faced in her young life. Whilst many children of 10 are able to talk with great clarity about their situation, Angela is not ready to do so. Counsellors of children such as Angela need to live with the uncertainty of not knowing 'the facts' and respond skilfully to what is present.

4 Become a safe container

It is necessary to be calm and confident in allowing Angela to be silent and play in her own way. To become anxious or insistent would add to Angela's fears.

5 Stop if you feel the child is genuinely not benefiting from the play

When Angela returns for session two, she is able to speak about the play. She makes many play dough cakes that are baked in an imaginary oven. She wants new play dough cutters for the next session and is obviously looking forward to more counselling 'play'. She is benefiting, though the sense of fear and uncertainty remain. It is early days.

There is more exploration of skilful play in counselling in Chapter 7. Levine's principles are based on research into the physiology and psychology of trauma. The straightforward steps he outlines where, in some ways, less is more, can enable counsellors to form relationships with traumatised children.

When trauma is present, it is likely that the young client will relate to their counsellor in an atypical manner for their age. In Angela's case, the way she plays would be more typical of a child aged 5 or 6. This behaviour gives lots of clues as to Angela's issues. Asking her specific questions about her life circumstances before there is a relationship established would bring about withdrawal and Angela would probably not attend counselling again. We can learn to recognise trauma and respond appropriately, whether that means continuing with counselling as outlined above or referring our young client to a specialised service.

Elements of Levine's approach can be applied to all children or young people with whom there are challenges when forming a therapeutic relationship. A young client does not need to show signs of trauma to benefit.

The therapeutic alliance is central when counselling young clients. Westergaard (2013) explored counsellors' perspectives on 'what works when counselling young people'. In this study, 'building an effective relationship' was considered paramount by counsellors, regardless of their theoretical orientation.

In cases where trauma is present, the young client might not wish to discuss the traumatic events. There is no need to focus on a painful past and it may be counterproductive to do so. Allow young clients to decide when they are ready to talk about any issue.

CHAPTER SUMMARY

The beginning of the counselling journey with children and young people is a crucial time. We need to be skilful in our initial approach.

Skills for establishing a relationship

- Be 'mindful', taking breaks between clients, pacing not rushing and noticing bodily sensations, thoughts and feelings as they arise (see Chapter 3 on mindful presence).
- Be self-aware: know how you are in the counselling relationship. Are you comfortable or uncomfortable with a young client? For example, are you influenced by their dress, smell, accent or a likeness to someone else?
- Notice non-judgementally: it doesn't help to tell yourself you 'should' be someone other than who you are. If, for example, you are upset by self-harm, swearing or the vulnerability of a young child in difficult life circumstances, acknowledge this and talk to a colleague or supervisor or get further training.
- Remember that you were a child and an adolescent once and there is a part of you that can join with a young person. Your inner child can be stimulated when establishing a counselling relationship with a child. This can bring joy and fun to the counselling room or other strong emotions such as sadness and regret.

H.E.A.R.O.S.:

- Holding the overview
- Empathy
- Age-appropriateness
- Resilience
- Openness to difference
- Self-care

- Take into account the age of clients and the ways in which you can expect them to respond according to their development.
- Consider individuality and not making assumptions concerning 'types' of clients.
- Notice if a young client appears disturbed or very frightened – there could be trauma or mental health issues present and they may respond in a manner that is atypical for their age.
- Remember that self-care is a necessary part of building the resilience required to begin the counselling journey with children and young people.

REFERENCES

Bowlby, J. (1988) *A Secure Base: Clinical Applications of Attachment Theory*. London: Routledge.
Erikson, E. (1995) *Childhood and Society*. London: Vintage.

Geldard, K. and Geldard, D. (2010) *Counselling Adolescents*. London: Sage.

Kabat-Zinn, J. (2003) 'Mindfulness-based interventions in context: past, present and future', *Clinical Psychology: Science and Practice*, 10(2): 144–56.

Kohlberg, L. (1984) *The Psychology of Moral Development*. San Francisco, CA: Harper & Row.

Levine, P. (2010) *In an Unspoken Voice*. Berkeley, CA: North Atlantic Books.

Piaget, J. (2001) *The Psychology of Intelligence*. London: Routledge Classics.

Rothschild, B. (2006) *The Body Remembers*. New York: W.W. Norton.

Stewart, I. and Joines, V. (2012) *TA Today: A New Introduction to Transactional Analysis*, 2nd edn. Chapel Hill, NC: Lifespace Publishing.

Weiss, L. (1999) *The Therapist's Guide to Self-Care*. London: Brunner Routledge.

Westergaard, J. (2013) 'Counselling young people: counsellors' perspectives on "what works" – an exploratory study', *Counselling and Psychotherapy Research*, 13(2): 98–105.

2

ASSESSING A YOUNG CLIENT

INTRODUCTION

Counsellors are often asked to measure outcomes and use assessment and evaluation procedures with young clients. How we approach these measurements can set the tone of counselling. We may find that making a therapeutic alliance and 'form filling' don't always fit together easily.

Monitoring counselling is necessary when clients are children and young people to ensure safety, accountability and maintenance of standards. We also need to show others that counselling services work well for children and young people.

We can develop our skills for assessing young clients; not relying solely on outcome measurements, rather combining them with our own knowing and the client's self-assessment.

In this chapter:

- Dilemmas in assessment
- Skills in completing forms
- Clients' suitability for counselling
- Including adults in assessment processes
- Assessing our ability to counsel a young client

DILEMMAS IN ASSESSMENT

There are some lines in a song that identify the dilemma that counsellors face when implementing assessment procedures with young clients: 'Inch worm, inch worm, measuring the marigolds seems to me you'll stop and see how beautiful they are' (Loesser 1951).

Children and young people are endlessly diverse and often bring to the counselling room a 'freshness', a new viewpoint, an innocence, a sense of fun and a less 'jaded' outlook on life. These are qualities that can be said to be immeasurable. Children are sometimes compared to opening flower buds. Whilst it is necessary to be realistic and not romanticise childhood, it can be troubling for counsellors and feel like an imposition if assessment processes are found to be demanding and do not fit with the agenda the young client brings to the counselling room.

Assessment and counselling

Counsellors are trained in empathy, joining with the client and enabling people through relationship, as we saw in Chapter 1. Many forms of assessment are clinical and use number to measure levels of risk, well-being and state of mind. Assessment and counselling are two different skills.

> ### MINDFUL MOMENT: ASSESSMENT AND COUNSELLING IN YOU
>
> Place two cushions on the floor in front of you. On one cushion imagine the aspect of yourself that is an assessor; on the second cushion, the aspect that is a counsellor. Take a moment to breathe and stop.
>   Notice what arises as you place your attention first on one cushion and then the other. What is happening in your body? Do your breathing, posture or gesture change when you focus on the assessing aspect or the counselling aspect of yourself?
>   What are the qualities of the assessor? What are the qualities of the counsellor? Both may have helpful qualities for you to recognise and aspects you don't like. How do these two aspects of you relate to one another? Do they get on well? Are they complementary or do they conflict with each other? After a few minutes, stop again, just breathe and allow these two aspects to integrate into you in a way that feels comfortable for you.
>   Note down your responses and consider how they may affect you when you are asked to assess young clients. You may want to bring your findings to a trusted colleague or your supervisor.

Responses to assessment

Older children and adolescents may have strong feelings and opinions about assessment, some enjoying it like a 'quiz', others finding it irrelevant or inappropriate. Young people spend a great deal of time being measured at school each day; this may mean they have a familiarity with being assessed that helps the process or it may mean there is a resentment, a sense of being judged. Younger clients may not understand assessment processes, requiring us to either complete assessments on their behalf or help them to do so.

Methods of assessing

It is valuable for counsellors to become adept and skilful in methods of assessing children and young people.

For professionals in other helping professions working with the young, detailed assessment is central to understanding how best to meet the young client's needs. Factors such as early attachment, current environmental situation and medical diagnoses will influence how a client is viewed just as much and often more than what the client wants, says or does.

Counsellors also need to understand how a child's early life or home circumstances are affecting them, consider any medical diagnosis or current medication and recognise any risk factors present. For counsellors, however, the young client's self-assessment will be important and central during counselling. Children and young people, given the opportunity, can be insightful into what they want and need to change in their lives, even at a very young age. As adults, we hold an awareness of how our young clients' stage of development will affect their choices and understanding of their life situation. This was explored in Chapter 1.

Counsellors need to respect how their young clients assess the situation they are in. Adults can be dismissive of children's opinions. A child who tells an adult they hate their mum or can't stand their geography lesson may be told that it is 'wrong to say that' by adults in their lives. Counsellors take a client-centred view and accept a child's feelings and opinions. This client-centred approach needs to be applied to assessment in counselling. Assessment should not be imposed on young clients.

SKILLS IN COMPLETING ASSESSMENT 'FORMS'

Assessment tends to be part of the framework of counselling, rather than part of the therapeutic relationship. On first meeting a young client, you may notice certain behaviour or sense an atmosphere of, for example, extreme anxiety. If, at that point, you carry out an assessment procedure with your client, you may find that the answers given on the form filled in by the client match what you have been noticing about their behaviour. Sometimes, however, the results of filling in forms differ widely from counsellors' perceptions of young clients. How then can 'form-based' assessment be skilfully used when counselling children and young people?

There are assessment tools that use scales and multiple-choice answers. These can provide quantitative data that can easily be translated into evidence understood in the wider community outside of psychotherapy and counselling. Commonly, counsellors of the young working in agencies or institutions will be required to implement a form-based assessment showing how the young client presents at the beginning of the counselling and then implement another assessment near the end of counselling to show if measurable change has taken place.

Some counsellors will be familiar with using forms and measurement in their initial training; for others, assessments that require bringing in an agenda that is not from the client's presenting issues can be alien and objectionable. More will be said about these differences when we consider modalities of initial training in Chapter 4.

As counsellors of the young, it is necessary to recognise that most clients do not have the means to pay. Counselling needs to be funded if it is to reach a majority of children and young people, rather than only a small minority of youngsters whose families can afford to pay for their counselling. Those who fund counselling want to know that there are useful outcomes from counselling children and young people. Gaining this knowledge involves assessment and the evaluation of services being carried out. For counsellors and young clients too, assessment can be useful and empowering. Young clients expressing their own views concerning how well the counselling service is working for them can be considered client-centred evaluation.

Approaching assessment – wise mind

Counsellors can enable 'form-based' assessment processes by neither treating them as 'the answer to everything' nor rejecting and objecting to them. Many helping professionals are overburdened with paperwork. Feeling 'burdened' by assessment paperwork or computer time is the experience of some counsellors working with young clients. Assessment can involve a great deal of time and effort, some of it outside the time of the counselling session. However, it is necessary to gain experience of using assessment forms and to be skilled and relaxed in using them, especially if they are a requirement of the agency which is employing the counsellor. This approach is the best we can offer young clients who will quite often be more 'at home' with form-based assessment than their counsellors, being from a different generation and growing up in a technological age. Marsha Linehan (Linehan and Lungu 2012) offers us the concept of the 'wise mind' as the place where the 'reasonable mind' and the 'emotional mind' integrate, enabling us to include analysis, observation, experience and intuition in decision making. Counsellors can approach the process of assessing clients by engaging their 'wise mind'.

If we just use a form and take the 'score', accepting tick-box answers alone to represent the young client and what their condition is, we may be denying the evidence of our emotional mind and finely tuned awareness honed and developed in training and practice. If we assess using our intuition and feeling about a client alone, there could easily be bias and assumptions made based on previous cases or on whom the client reminds us of. When the two types of knowing are combined, a place of skill and balance can be found within the assessment process.

YP CORE, an outcome measure

YP CORE (from CORE Information Management Systems) is a widely used 'outcome measure' – a method of assessing risk and levels of change. The form has just ten items and is 'user-friendly' for the majority of 11–16-year-olds (to see the form, visit the CORE ims website at www.coreims.co.uk).

When used alongside an 'intake' form used for statistical information and other forms to show a young client's pattern of attendance at counselling, it amounts to plenty of paperwork for the counsellor!

The outcome measure offers two reasons for its use as explanations that counsellors can give to young clients about the procedure:

- to help us better understand the problems you wish to address in counselling
- to help us directly in our work with you and to help us learn how best to improve our services. (YP CORE user manual V1-23)

As there are ten multiple-choice items on YP CORE, the first of these reasons will be relevant for some clients and not for others whose specific problem may not be represented in YP CORE.

The following case example illuminates the challenges in designing a measurement system that works across any client group. It offers counsellors the opportunity to use their 'wise mind' when assessing and using outcome measures.

CASE EXAMPLE: HARRY FILLS IN A FORM

Harry is 12 and enthusiastically approaches the forms he is given to fill in. There are ten items and they each have four multiple-choice answers. For most of the items, a score of 4 shows the highest level of problem in functioning. Harry fills in the questionnaire attentively and when you look at his answers you realise he has scored zero for each – a score of zero suggests he is fine and has done everything that he wants to do this week. You are counselling Harry in a school and the school staff have informed you that if Harry says he has seen his mother you must disclose this. Harry is in the care of his grandfather and not allowed by law to see his mother unaccompanied. If his mother comes to the school, the police must be called. Harry's drawings suggest he feels both disturbed and very isolated. He draws himself as a tiny figure on one half of the paper and everyone else as tiny figures in the distance.

Limitations of multiple choice

This example shows the limitations of multiple choice in using outcome measures. Even when the counsellor uses the outcome measure again with Harry in a later session, explaining the questions to make sure he has understood, the results are exactly the same. Harry is benefiting from the counselling, he enjoys the sessions, engages in activities in the counselling room and there is a relationship developing between client and counsellor. Possibly, one day, Harry will be scoring more highly on the multiple choice items. Would this mean he is 'getting worse'? More likely, it would mean that Harry's self-awareness level had changed and grown. At the moment, anything Harry feels about not being in contact with his mother and the events that led up to this are either out of his awareness or denied. Harry has told the counsellor that he 'doesn't like to think about' the events that led up to his enforced separation from his mother.

This must be respected and may be the best option for Harry at this time. If he was judged according to his numerical score, very little useful information could be gained. The counsellor then uses 'wise mind' and makes a case for continuing to counsel Harry despite his zero score.

The answers on multiple-choice forms of this kind can be fed into a computer to gain statistical analysis. Harry's 'score' may not be statistically significant to the outcomes of data collected from young clients. The majority of young clients are offering scores that can be measured and give useful results. Mick Cooper (2008) tells us that the 'facts are friendly'. Research into counselling shows that it works.

Funding that enables counselling services for children and young people to exist can be contingent on the statistics showing good outcomes. For many young people's counsellors, form filling is an inevitable part of the work. YP CORE was designed in consultation with young people. Researchers found that 'the brevity of measure ensures that young people do not find its completion too onerous' (Twigg et al. 2009: 166). The great majority of young clients will manage YP CORE and other straightforward outcome measures well. As counsellors, we can be the gatekeepers of these types of measurements, recognising the few occasions where their use is either inappropriate or of limited value.

Creative means with multiple-choice forms

Some counsellors and clients find very creative ways of managing forms. Graphs, for example, showing where anxiety scores have reduced can be enjoyed by the young person. Sometimes young clients have forgotten that they scored so highly on anxiety in the past and feel delighted when they realise that their anxiety has reduced so much. It is crucial that the young client is not judged by their score alone: 'She's high risk, she scored 35' can be a helpful statement only in the context of double checking and trusting our knowledge of the client gained through relationship with them.

Statistical analysis is just one kind of assessment and some counsellors of children and young people might find that other types of assessment are far more relevant to their practice.

Assessment from others

When counselling younger children, questions may arise as to other people's assessment of the child, not what the child feels or thinks about their own situation. Counsellors may have information about a child's situation that the child doesn't have. Counselling a child in foster care who has contact with one parent is an example of this. The child is waiting to 'go home', but you have been told that a complex legal situation means that this child is unlikely to be allowed to live with their parent. What the child thinks and wants is directly opposed to what is happening in their life. The challenging part for the counsellor is in knowing the facts but being told it's in the best interests of the client not to know the facts about their own life. For a client-centred practitioner, this involves managing a dilemma and the situation will need to be regularly discussed in supervision.

Balancing confidentiality and feedback to others

If we are asked to assess a child we are counselling and give information to others (parents, teachers, social workers, etc.), how do we go about this ethically, balancing our duty of confidentiality with others' need to know about the child?

There is certain useful information we can give whilst maintaining confidentiality. We can:

- confirm that our young client is engaging in counselling processes
- express any concerns about a need for further help from other agencies
- explain likely behaviour changes in a given set of circumstances.

This can all be done without breaking the young client's confidentiality. Unlike counselling adults, it is often not possible to keep the fact that children are attending counselling confidential.

An example of this is Janna, aged 9, who confides in you that she is upset as her brother is always 'right' according to how her parents view family situations. It would be a betrayal of trust to repeat what Janna had said about her parents to them; however, saying to the parents that Janna is making very good use of the counselling or facilitating a meeting between Janna and her parents where she expresses some of her feelings and says what she would like to be different at home could be an appropriate use of the counsellor's role. It is so important not to either lose sight of the young person's perspective or collude with them against their parents and teachers. Counsellors have a unique opportunity to enter 'non-judgementally' into the lives of children and young people and need to manage those instances where something may not be to their personal taste but is reasonable parenting or teaching. It is for this reason that checking out 'causes for concern' in supervision is part of the assessment of young clients.

ASSESSING SUITABILITY FOR COUNSELLING

First contact with the client

An initial meeting or telephone discussion with the adult responsible for referring a young client to counselling often provides the first information counsellors receive. This in itself leads to a dilemma: how much do we want to know about our clients before we meet them? Can we accept the information a referring adult gives us and still keep an open mind when meeting a new client?

REFLECTIVE ACTIVITY

Using this reflection as a journal entry or in discussion with colleagues, consider the effect the following information has on you, which is given to you before meeting a young client:

- Mary's mum died in a car crash five years ago. Mary, now 17, was in the car but was uninjured.
- Luke, 9, is on medication for ADHD (Attention Deficit Hyperactivity Disorder).
- Josh, 6, is the younger brother of Adam who you saw for counselling last year at his school.
- Ahmed, 15, has had leukaemia.
- Kristina is 12, her parents have separated and her father moved away recently.
- There are concerns about Hugh being neglected; he seems tired and hungry and his clothes are dirty.
- Kate is such a lovely, bubbly girl and good at most subjects in school, so we can't understand why she is truanting.

How do you think being given this kind of information about a young client might affect your first meeting with them?

We may need to have information like this and find it helpful. It is, however, necessary to consider what we will do if our client doesn't talk to us about what we now know, having been told by a referring adult. Do you discuss what you have been told about your client with them in counselling?

In some cases, it is not ethical to refer to information you have been given elsewhere. You cannot tell Josh (above) that you have seen his older brother for counselling previously as this would break his brother's confidential agreement with you. In other situations, you may want to bring to counselling the information you have been given. How is it best to do this?

CASE EXAMPLE: RECEIVING INFORMATION ABOUT YOUR CLIENT

Kristina, your new client, comes to counselling not knowing that you have already been given some information about her by a youth worker in a discussion you had. You are told: 'Kristina has changed since her dad left.'

Kristina is a 12-year-old who looks 16; she is tall, has the figure of a young woman and is wearing make-up, heels and fashionable clothes. This is her first experience of counselling and she sweeps into the counselling room, flicking her hair into shape and adjusting her skirt as she sits down. She smiles and speaks to you during this first session about not getting on with her friends and being 'grounded' by her mum. She does not mention her parents' situation at all. Would you bring to counselling the knowledge that you have concerning the separation?

You have been told by the youth worker that Kristina's father has recently left the family home, but Kristina doesn't mention this. The situation leaves you with a dilemma that needs to be handled skilfully to make the best choice.

Sometimes young people presume that the counsellor knows all about their past and current circumstances. Sharing information is the 'norm' in children's lives and is often good practice as professionals work together on behalf of the child or young person. Young clients can, however, express shock, embarrassment or resentment when information held by the counsellor about them is introduced into the privacy of the counselling room.

Reasons for sharing what you know with Kristina:

- You can check for accuracy of the youth worker's information. Kristina's dad may have been very distant from her before the separation and his leaving may make little difference to her day-to-day life or he may have been a vital part of her life, a loving dad, and she is experiencing great loss. Clarifying with her could be a useful part of gaining trust and she may feel relieved that you know.

- If you know something about Kristina that she doesn't know you know, this can interfere with your ability to get to know her. The knowledge is 'in the room' and unspoken. You might be left wondering why Kristina didn't tell you if she doesn't mention it at all.

Reasons for *not* sharing what you know with Kristina:

- Kristina may genuinely not want or need to talk about her dad leaving. Right now her problem is how she is not getting on with her mum. She may feel puzzled or even offended if you bring in knowledge about her given to you by others.

- Kristina may assume (wrongly) that you are going to talk with others about her again because you have done so once. Her privacy is so important to her that any conversation between adults where she is discussed is not OK with her.

Choosing whether to share information with your client

Choosing when and if to talk to 'Kristina' or any young client about information you have been given concerning them is not simple. There are differing factors to take into consideration in each case. Some skills can be applied that fit most cases. The first action is to consult your clinical supervisor if you are in doubt, as talking this through may enable a clear choice to be made without delay. In making the decision whether to share or 'disclose' what you know, the following skills will be helpful:

Timing

Choose your moment with care. If a client is very distressed, then the current circumstances will be the priority and it is not appropriate to bring in referral information. If the client is not very distressed and you sense the need to say what you have been told, then it is useful to say, for example:

> Someone [name the person if possible] has given me this information about you. I don't yet know if that's what you want to talk about, or if it is how you understand what is happening in your life. We will talk only about what you want to bring to counselling whilst we are together each week; I just need to check this information out with you to be clear about your current life situation.

This statement would be accompanied by a 'safety' clause in the contract (contracting will be covered in Chapter 5) where it is made clear at the outset what can and cannot stay completely confidential.

This early intervention can avoid the situation where you want to mention something you have been told about your client to them, but find it more difficult and complex to introduce once counselling is under way. The initial session is 'getting to know each other' time and explaining what you already know fits best there.

Context

Be clear with your young client that the type of conversation that takes place outside of counselling where you listen to what other professionals or parents/carers say about them will happen rarely. Tell your client that you will *only listen* and will not disclose the subject matter of the counselling to others. You will not be sharing information with anyone else unless there is risk of significant harm or your client has requested that you do so (see Chapter 5).

Advocacy

It is possible that a client will ask you to share information they have given to you in counselling with others and sometimes this is appropriate. An 'advocacy' role can be part of the work of a counsellor with children and young people.

Passing on information to the youth worker that a client such as Kristina might need 'time out', a chance to cool off when there is conflict in school or family life, will give her a voice, an ally in communicating with the adult world. Permission from your young client to share information on their behalf is vital. Counsellors can never be sure how information passed on will be used.

When counselling younger children, factual conversations about why a child is behaving differently or 'badly' can be helpful. If, for example, a parent has been ill or a big change in home circumstances has occurred, explaining to adults that a child's reactions are understandable and common in response to the current circumstances can be useful.

Counselling or not?

Now we have met the new client for the first time, there is a process of deciding if the client's best interests are served by attending counselling. It seems likely that a client such as Kristina in the case study above would benefit from being in counselling. Other potential clients will have a less obvious need or desire to be counselled. Troubled children and young people are often a great challenge to their parents/carers and teachers; if a counsellor is available then there can be a 'magic wand' approach as if sending the child to counselling will be the cure for all their problems. Whilst there are many occasions when counselling will be beneficial, there are some circumstances where it will not be the correct intervention. Counsellors need skills to either purposefully accept young clients or know when and how to refer on, deciding that counselling is not the right way forward in a given situation.

In the right place?

Young clients who arrive in the counselling room are not always in the right place. Counsellors need to learn to assess professionally and confidently and to only accept a client *if* it is in that client's best interests to do so.

Other professionals have definite, fixed criteria for accepting a young client. Child and adolescent mental health services, for example, will often assess and decide against admitting a young person, even though there are clearly serious problems in their lives, if the young person does not fit their admissions criteria.

Counsellors may accept most of the children and young people that arrive for counselling as they have a client-centred approach and an openness to forming a relationship to enable change but there are limitations for counsellors too on who can be accepted as a client.

The caring nature of counsellors working with the young means that sometimes a client is accepted into counselling when it is not appropriate simply because there are no other options for them to get the help they need. Discussing cases in supervision can bring to light a concern in the counsellor that the client is not benefiting in any way and may be avoiding something else by coming to counselling. Misbehaving in school, for example, can be a reason for referring a child or young person to a counsellor. This may be an appropriate referral as long as everyone concerned understands that it is not the counsellor's task to make the child behave differently in their lessons.

We must be clear about assessing who is suitable for counselling, even though we hope to reach out to a wide range of young people and not exclude anyone unnecessarily.

Counsellors assess young clients' suitability for counselling in a variety of ways. These include:

- connecting through intuition and presence, recognising if psychological contact has been made
- listening carefully and responding appropriately to the client as an individual
- noticing behaviour in the counselling room
- recognising own feelings and thoughts and how responses to a particular client may affect the counselling
- considering risk factors and making decisions about how to proceed
- identifying the issues that can be addressed in counselling
- discussing with clinical supervisor if doubts or concerns about the young client's suitability for counselling arise.

These are just a selection of the skills that counsellors employ in making an assessment of young clients. Counsellors are trained to have high levels of awareness and using this awareness is an integral part of how assessment is carried out.

These are vital skills for counsellors and will be considered fully later in the next chapter on essential counselling skills. Here, the focus is on making the best choice for the potential young client. Is beginning counselling with you a good option for them at this time?

Accepting a young client for counselling

When deciding whether or not to accept a child or young person for counselling, what do counsellors need to take into account?

Counsellors may offer an assessment or introductory session before starting the counselling process. This may be a requirement of the agency or the choice of the counsellor. How the assessment session is carried out can set the tone for what is to follow.

It is necessary to use some different skills when assessing to those you use during regular counselling.

During assessment:

1. Keep focused on the information you need to gain in order to make the assessment.
2. Explain that this may be the only time you meet and you are here to find out if counselling is the right way to help.
3. Allow the young client to assess 'counselling' by asking any questions they may have.

INCLUDING ADULTS IN REFERRAL PROCESSES

With younger clients who are unlikely to be competent to make decisions about attending counselling, you may include the adult who has referred them in part or all of the assessment. There are various ways to do this:

1 Speak to the adult whilst the young client is in a waiting room

This is recommended only in occasional circumstances where there are few options. It may happen in private practice when there has been no opportunity to speak to the referrer in advance. Generally, leaving the young client in the waiting room is not to be recommended. It is, however, preferable to talking about the young person when they are present 'as if' they were not there. An example of this is the parent who brings a child to the first session and, at the door, before you have even sat down begins to tell you 's/he has always been a bit of a scatterbrain' or 's/he is a little monster'. This situation needs to be prevented and speaking to the parent alone briefly may be the best way to do this. This is provided the child is of an age that they could be safely and happily occupied in a suitable waiting room.

2 Speak to the adult on the phone before the first session

Often, a parent or carer will phone and want to tell you the 'problem'. It is a good idea to listen, remembering that if the young client is seen as 'the problem' in a family situation, this is unlikely to be the same story as the one that will be told to you by the young client later when you meet them. You may hear what narrative therapists call a 'thin description'. This is a description that offers a very narrow reason for the young client's behaviour. Morgan (undated) gives the case example of Sean who, his family believes, won't stop stealing because he is an attention seeker. It is useful not to form any opinion of young clients based on this type of initial conversation. We can, of course, empathise with any parent or carer who is finding a child or young person 'difficult'. It is helpful to have a good relationship with the person who is bringing a young client to counselling. This early contact with the referrer is useful for sorting out practical issues like who pays for the counselling and how payment will be made.

3 Adult comes into introductory session

It can be a good idea to talk to the adult with the young client present. Issues of confidentiality (discussed in Chapter 5) can be usefully discussed with both adult and young client early in the first session. The counsellor needs to be holding the 'boundaries' in this situation: welcoming the young client and explaining to them that you will not be sharing the contents of the session with anyone unless there is a risk of harm. This is usefully done with the adult in the room.

If adults cannot accept the confidentiality agreement, it is good to know this as early as possible in the process.

4 Assess the young client first, confirm arrangements with adult

This is a good strategy with older children, those who are 'Gillick competent'. Adolescent clients particularly appreciate being treated with respect and being spoken to directly. It is good practice to check out with young clients before speaking to referrers at all, even if it is only to confirm transport arrangements for the next session. Counsellors will need to decide, based on the age of the potential client and the context of the counselling, which of the above ways of managing the first session are most appropriate.

Create an information sheet for parents/carers explaining what counselling will entail and how any information the parent/carer needs will be given.

INFORMATION SHEET: KEY ISSUES FOR PARENTS/CARERS/ OTHER REFERRING ADULTS

WHAT IS COUNSELLING?

Counselling is the opportunity to talk about things that are of concern, to a child or young person, in confidence, with a qualified counsellor. What is spoken about will depend on the individual, but common themes are stress, relationships, change, loss and distressing, traumatic events.

WHAT DOES A COUNSELLOR DO?

Counsellors are trained to listen without judging and to help people sort out their thoughts and feelings about whatever is concerning them.

A key feature of our service is that information discussed in the counselling session is treated confidentially. Counselling is a time when it's OK to talk about concerns without fear of them being discussed elsewhere. This includes not discussing the work with parents, carers or other adults unless the child or young person requests or gives consent for this. This can be hard to accept at times, but ensuring confidentiality of the work is crucial for establishing trust so that children and young people feel confident to speak openly and freely about what is concerning them.

However, if a child appears to be at risk of significant harm it may be appropriate to seek help from other agencies to keep them safe. The counsellor would aim to discuss this first with the child or young person concerned. All counsellors receive supervision of their work with young people, to ensure the quality of their practice. *(Adapted from BACP/WAG (undated))*

Many of the issues raised here, particularly those concerning confidentiality and supervision, are addressed in later chapters in the book.

Questions for the counsellor

These are some questions you can ask to enable best practice in assessing a young person coming into counselling:

- Has the young client agreed to come to counselling?
- Is the client bringing an issue that can be addressed by the counselling process?
- Is it within the range of the counsellor's skills and experience to counsel this particular young person?
- Do this particular client's issues raise any practical dilemmas for the counsellor?
- What will we do next if a client seems unsuitable for counselling? (Consider referral procedures, skilful ways to refer on, what to say to parents/carers and teachers.)

Has the young client agreed to come to counselling?

The question of agreeing to be counselled is one that arises rarely with adult clients, but often with children and young people, many of whom have not agreed to come to counselling and do not have much information about what counselling is. Self-referral will usually be limited to adolescents who have been introduced to the counselling process. Children can be referred to counselling when they have not requested to come because they are showing symptoms or have situations in their lives that concern the adults around them. These include:

- behavioural problems
- family problems
- disagreements with parents/carers or teachers
- changes in school attendance or grades
- divorce or separation of parents
- symptoms of depression and/or anxiety
- anger management.

Young people whose problem behaviour is affecting others may be sent to counselling. This seems like a useful answer for the adults who are responsible for them. To the young person, it may be confusing and worrying as young people can be 'scapegoats' in difficult family situations. It needs to be made clear to the potential client that you do not immediately believe what you are told by others. You want to hear the client's story and then make a choice about how to proceed that is in the best interests of the client.

Can the client make good use of counselling even though they have not agreed to attend initially? Recent research has suggested that outcomes of counselling with young clients can be successful, whether young clients choose to come to counselling or are sent. So what is it that the counsellor is assessing?

The initial session with the client Describe what counselling is. Explain that we are not going to try and 'persuade' them to behave differently. Our task is not to punish, tell off, be disappointed in their behaviour or make them do their homework.

Inviting questions Once the young client knows this to be true and it needs to be true in action as well as in words, then the counsellor can begin to assess whether the client is able to engage in counselling despite not choosing to come. It is not possible to continue to counsel if there is a genuine desire in the young client to 'escape' from the counselling. Reluctance, however, can be due to a lack of understanding of what counselling is. Some youngsters just do not want to talk about their lives and counselling is probably not for them, no matter how much we or other adults believe it would help.

Listening with an open mind Assessment begins with listening, an open mind and the humility to admit you don't have any way of knowing what is actually happening until you get to know your client.

CASE EXAMPLE: A 15-YEAR-OLD 'TOLD' TO COME TO COUNSELLING

Mario has stopped going to school. He is 15 and refuses to attend any alternative arrangements made for him to study. He lives with his mother who hardly sees him as he stays with older friends in town. He wants to attend the local drop-in centre for 16–25-year-olds. The manager of the centre is concerned about Mario and does not want him to be out on the streets but recognises he should, in fact, be in school. An arrangement is made that Mario can attend the drop-in centre if he goes to counselling. The manager of the drop-in centre asks you to counsel Mario. You have your doubts about the suitability of Mario for counselling. You agree to see him and talk to him about what counselling is. Mario agrees to see you because he wants to be allowed into the drop-in centre.

Congruence is needed to gain trust with Mario. If he tells you that he is only coming to counselling because he wants to attend the drop-in centre, how do you respond to this in order to try and begin the therapeutic alliance?

Possible responses

◆ Parental: 'That's not a good reason; please consider why else you might need to come' will mean Mario views you as just one of those adults who are trying to control him and make him do something he does not want to do.

- ◆ Joining with the adolescent: accessing your inner adolescent so that you can 'join' with Mario's style of communication will help the assessment process (Geldard and Geldard 2010). We also need to remember our responsible position as counsellors whilst joining with the adolescent. More will be written on this in the counselling skills chapter that follows.

Some options of how to respond to Mario include:

- ◆ 'It's a challenge but let's see if we can make it work for both of us.'
- ◆ 'So you are only here because counselling is the key to the drop-in centre … do you want to give counselling a try then?'
- ◆ 'You don't like to be told what to do and that suits me 'cos it's my job to find out what you want.'

If Mario responds positively to any of these, saying he will give counselling a try, then make a start!

For adolescents to make use of counselling, there is a need for them to accept some responsibility for the 'problems' they face.

Young children, inevitably, are subject to the will, rules and choices of adults who are responsible for them, and sometimes the issues in their lives are not of their own making at all. Even in cases where problems are caused completely by adults, there is a place for counselling to enable children to comprehend, for example, that they are not the 'bad' child that they have been labelled.

Similarly to the case of Mario above, a 15-year-old comes to counselling. Karla has come voluntarily, but with an 'agenda' that needs to be carefully considered.

CASE EXAMPLE: KARLA HAS BEEN ARRESTED

Karla, aged 15, comes to counselling in her local youth centre because she has been arrested for shoplifting. Her legal representative has advised counselling. Karla is worried about being caught and prosecuted but not concerned at all about the action of shoplifting, viewing it only as 'a laugh'. Karla thinks it might help her in court if she says she attended counselling. As the counselling session begins, she tells you she is 'fine' and just fed up with her friends who didn't run fast enough when the shop assistant caught them.

If there is a general understanding that counselling is a method of getting sympathy from the legal profession, then it makes the counselling difficult but not impossible. Some young people will find they engage in the counselling process

(Continued)

> *(Continued)*
>
> even if this was not their initial intention. The counsellor needs to maintain an open mind and be aware too that there may be a request from the court to get a professional opinion as to the character of the young client. You may find that Karla begins to talk about her life; if so, counselling can begin. Her arrival in the counselling room does not mean she is engaged in counselling and you may need to explain this to Karla or any young client with a similar agenda.

Rogers (1961, cited in Tolan 2012) identified seven stages of the process, where a client can move from a rigid world view where outcomes are the 'fault' of others and there is a belief that change is impossible, towards a more fluid view of the world with acceptance of personal responsibility. It is recognised that people in Rogers' stages one or two, where problems are identified as someone else's fault or created by other people, would be unlikely to seek counselling (Tolan 2012).

Young people in these early stages of the process, such as Mario or Karla above, will, however, arrive in the counselling room because they have been sent or told by others that it will help with a problem such as a court case.

Those who are not ready to change at all, say they are 'fine' or don't want to talk about what is going on in their lives and feel that problems are never of their making are not good candidates for counselling at this point in their lives. They can be invited to come back to counselling later and treated in a compassionate and respectful manner, but it needs to be recognised that counselling cannot help right now.

To assess whether Karla or young people in a similar situation to her are actually interested in counselling at all, the following procedure can be used:

- Explain clearly what counselling is and who you are in 'young people friendly' language.

- Be clear that s/he needs to 'engage' with you for you to be able to do your job. This will involve talking, drawing, playing or being together in a manner that enables reflection, thinking and/or expressing feelings about actions in their own life that have brought them to counselling.

- Say you are not going to judge, rather explore the whole situation and discover together if any change would enable a better approach to life.

- Maintain a level of self-respect and professionalism and do not be 'used' for ulterior motives, whether this is a court case or so that the young client can miss another activity such as double maths.

- Be open, friendly and interested in the initial reticence of a client, and this may enable their first experience of 'opening up' in the therapeutic process.

Introducing older children and adolescents to counselling in this way is particularly helpful.

The counsellor's skills and experience to counsel a particular young client

Trauma, mental health problems, severe behavioural problems and learning difficulties are issues that counsellors have to assess on an individual basis, case by case, before deciding whether to accept a young client into counselling. The 'fit' between counsellor and client needs to be considered. There is often not a clear yes or no answer.

Sometimes the counsellor is not ready to take on a very distressed young child showing signs of trauma, finding the work too upsetting. However, another counsellor might be able to counsel this child. Aggressive adolescents can be an enjoyable challenge for some counsellors, whilst for others the challenge is not appealing in any way and can be both frightening and deskilling.

> **CASE EXAMPLE: ANDY'S NIGHTMARES**
>
> Andy is sent to see you because he is suffering from nightmares and not sleeping. He is your first appointment that day at 9.30 am. He is 17 and discloses to you that he has smoked 'dope' and has had a few 'white-outs'. You begin to explore the situation with him and you sense a deep anxiety and confusion in him. He says that he feels that everyone is 'out to get him'. He tells you that he isn't sure what is real and what is 'in his head' anymore, and every so often during the counselling session he hits his own head with the flat of his hand and looks at you in a bewildered way. He asks you to repeat what you have just said a few times and seems to find it difficult being in counselling, saying it is too early in the day for him to focus.

Many issues arise from this first session with Andy. He has clearly broken the law and confidentiality dilemmas that arise will be discussed in Chapter 5.

This case also needs to be taken to supervision (see Chapter 8). What you choose to do next will partly depend on the context in which you are counselling Andy. There may be very clear actions that you need to take in referring Andy to a substance misuse agency that works with young people or to an adolescent mental health unit to assess his mental well-being. Andy needs to know the concerns you have about counselling him and that you would like to get other agencies involved with him.

It may, however, be the case that seeing Andy later in the day and making an agreement with him about not being under the influence of substances, even from the day before, when he comes to counselling will be enough to form a useful therapeutic relationship.

If the confusion and sense of paranoia continue to manifest in Andy, these symptoms suggest a mental health issue could be emerging. As counsellors, we need to be aware in assessment that this type of mental health issue often emerges in the teenage years. Whilst it is healthy to extend our range as counsellors, limitations need to be accepted and not seen as failures but as in the best interests of clients.

When deciding whether to accept a young client into counselling, consider:

Experience A client can be outside the range of our experience. A complex medical diagnosis with mental and physical health problems may require more specialist help.

Training Sometimes a counsellor needs further training to meet the needs of a young client in counselling. If the client has substance misuse issues, it is useful for us to know local terms for drugs and alcohol use and be aware of the likely consequences of trying different substances. This may require referral to a specialist agency.

Personal history A client having similar problems to those we have experienced can be either an advantage, if the problem has been addressed, or overwhelming and upsetting if not. An example of this is a counsellor who has experienced domestic violence. S/he could be highly appropriate for young clients who have a parent that has been violent. Alternatively, it may be too re-stimulating for the counsellor. If so, this is an issue for supervision at the earliest opportunity.

Current circumstances A counsellor who is divorcing may find young clients who are distressed by their parents' separation difficult to work with. If our current circumstances do impact in this way, don't just struggle on as support may be needed to manage this.

REFLECTIVE ACTIVITY: SKILLS IN ASSESSING YOUR SUITABILITY TO COUNSEL A CLIENT

Notice your anxiety if you feel out of your depth. Don't ignore worries and concerns.

- Make a personal list of signs and symptoms of being overstressed or re-stimulated by a young client's issues.
- Be aware that if you think about a client as you go to sleep or when you wake in the morning, these are clear warning signs.
- Plan actions you will take if you notice these symptoms.

You may be asked to see a child or young person who has difficulty engaging in counselling due to problems with their attention or ability to communicate with others or they may have been given medication for their condition. In this situation, it can be important that there is an opportunity for you to discuss the medical condition prior to counselling. There is sometimes little information concerning medical diagnoses given to counsellors in advance of the first counselling session. There is a need to be 'client-centred' and accept the young person who comes to counselling; it may be of real importance, however, to understand a medical issue or recent events in their life.

Practical dilemmas

Practical issues may arise when assessing whether to accept a young client into counselling with you. There may be issues concerning already being a counsellor to their sibling or girlfriend/boyfriend/best friend if we are counselling in a club, school or other youth agency. The potential new client may be the child of someone we know in the neighbourhood. It may seem clear to us that we would not counsel someone in these circumstances; however, if we are the only counsellor the young client can access, we may be denying them access to counselling they urgently need. Assessing each individual's circumstances is necessary before finally deciding whether or not to accept them into counselling.

In order to be able to make the best decision, we need to have a good idea of what else is available to support a potential client if we are not able to counsel them. We may be employed by an agency that gives us handbooks that include referral procedures; if so, be sure to read them and know what to do. It can be distressing for a counsellor to find themselves outside the limits of their competence, as described with Andy, and not know who to refer on to. It is possible to create a 'resource directory', which is likely to be a notebook. It could be developed online or on a smartphone or tablet, as it contains only agency and professional networking information.

Creating a resource directory A resource directory is a useful tool. It will include local information such as names and contact numbers of:

- your clinical supervisor
- the agency you work for
- the relevant link person (schools based)
- Child and Adolescent Mental Health Service (CAMHS)
- eating disorder helplines
- Childline
- bereavement help for children and young people including CRUSE and local organisations
- substance misuse agencies for young people.

Calling helplines There are many helplines where staff will be willing to talk to you in complete anonymity about a condition that a young client has. A specific circumstance may require a particular helpline not listed above. If a young client in their teens confides to you that they are not taking their medication regularly, you can encourage them to go back to their GP or tell their parent/carer. You may also wish to ring a specific helpline for that condition and talk through the consequences of erratic use of that prescribed substance. Sometimes not taking prescribed medication properly can be a serious issue requiring liaison with others to protect a young person from becoming very unwell.

Learn commonly used medical terms, so if you are told: 'She may have ADHD' (Attention Deficit Hyperactivity Disorder) or 'He is on the Autistic Spectrum', use your resource directory and you will either know what this means or how to find out. These terms are used often and it is good to have a working knowledge of how such conditions may present in the counselling room. Continuing professional development training or selected reading from reliable sources on the internet will help. The young client may be on medication for their condition and counsellors need to know how this may affect the counselling process, occasionally making the client unsuitable to be counselled.

When a client seems unsuitable for counselling

Making contact with the young client is vital for counselling to be possible. Young clients sometimes seem distant and distracted in the counselling room. Whilst some young clients are unsuitable for counselling, it is vital to take culture, language, gender, class and ability into consideration when deciding whether or not a client can be counselled.

Our own biases It is possible to unintentionally discriminate against a young client. Cultural biases need to be examined as we can miss a signal that a young client gives us because we are not familiar with their way of communicating. It may be that another counsellor would be more 'in tune' with a particular client, but that counsellor may not be available and we are then challenged to stretch our limits, confront our assumptions and explore our prejudices. Most, if not all, counsellors will be faced with this type of situation during their counselling practice. There may be an initial reaction or response that is based on our own life circumstances. Most counsellors will do their best to bring self-awareness to the assessment process before making decisions about a client's lack of suitability to be counselled. It is, however, necessary to recognise that it is possible to miss our own biases. An example given by Reid and Westergaard (2011) is noticing if we attribute certain behaviours to a group as 'natural'. They give the example of wrongly assuming that young people who are 'NEET' (not in education, employment or training) are 'not motivated' or 'cannot get up in the morning'. We may know that this is wrong thinking but there is still the possibility that we will, at times, make assumptions about young clients.

When counselling is not the right kind of help The client too may be reluctant to attend and, after one or two trial sessions, it could be necessary to advise the young client and whoever has referred them that the counselling is not going anywhere. It is important to maintain a 'no-blame' approach in this situation as youngsters who are experiencing the internal environment of counselling for the first time need to have the opportunity to come back if and when they want to do so. How many activities did we find boring and difficult as a teenager that we later came to enjoy?

Gardening, going for walks, eating long slow lunches, listening to talk radio, for example, can be boring to the young yet tremendously enjoyable later in life. Counselling and therapy might just have been offered at the wrong time or in an unacceptable way. Rebellion and determination to be different can make some adolescents resist it.

Sometimes, counselling is not the right kind of help and our task is to track down the right kind of help, from 'anger management' to a helpline or mentor. Referring on is a skill to be honed, possibly using the resource directory we create.

Using the BACP Ethical Framework The BACP Ethical Framework (2010) does not seek to hand out rules, but rather asks us to consider our practice and make the best possible choice in any given circumstances. Assessing whether to accept a client, or assessing whether it is ethical and legal to maintain confidentiality with that client (the subject of Chapter 6), is enabled through considering the principles of the BACP Ethical Framework.

The idea of competing principles, offered to counsellors in the BACP Ethical Framework, can be examined. Competing principles are often relevant to counsellors with young clients. There is often a need to decide whether the principle of 'beneficence' – a commitment to promoting the client's well-being – outweighs the principle of 'autonomy' – a respect for the client's right to be self-governing, when assessing issues in counselling children and young people. This will be addressed more fully in Chapter 6. Now, we are considering assessment and there are times when promoting a young client's well-being might include deciding whether counselling is the appropriate intervention. A child's sense of their own autonomy can be limited by the level of understanding they have of the consequences of their actions.

Finding a new perspective There is a story about a child looking out of the downstairs window of a house. The child looks frightened because the bushes are moving from side to side. A friendly adult asks the child what the problem is. The child replies: 'there is a monster in the bushes'. The adult takes the child by the hand and they go upstairs. Looking down on the same bush, two puppies can be seen playing. A new and different perspective has been gained, a new view. The child needed help to find this new perspective.

An assessment or an introductory session, skilfully implemented, can offer that new view. Even if problems are severe and insoluble, it may be possible to offer young clients support and a different way of understanding themselves in their life situation.

CHAPTER SUMMARY

- Be aware that being with children and young people in counselling and then assessing them can feel like a 'conflict' between two different sets of skills.
- Find the 'wise mind' approach that combines thinking and feeling about assessment.
- Use forms skilfully and confidently; don't, however, neglect relationship skills when assessing a young client.
- Assess suitability for counselling with an awareness of unintentional cultural biases and assumptions.

- Consider the impact of first contact with referring adults and how it may influence counselling.
- Use the BACP ethical principles and a methodical approach, taking into account:
    - the context
    - family relationships
    - a client's understanding of the counselling process and willingness to participate
    - any diagnosed condition the client has
    - any specific training you have received as a counsellor.

REFERENCES

British Association for Counselling and Psychotherapy (BACP) (2010) *Ethical Framework for Good Practice in Counselling and Psychotherapy*. Lutterworth: BACP.

BACP/Welsh Assembly Government (WAG) (undated) *Schools Based Counselling Operating ToolKit*. Available at: www.bacp.co.uk/crs/Ethics%20in%20Practice/schoolToolkit.php

Cooper, M. (2008) *Essential Findings in Counselling and Psychotherapy: The Facts are Friendly*. London: Sage.

Geldard, K. and Geldard, D. (2010) *Counselling Adolescents*. London: Sage.

Linehan, M. and Lungu, A. (2012) 'Compassion, wisdom and suicidal clients', in K. Germer and D. Siegel (eds), *Wisdom and Compassion in Psychotherapy, Deepening Mindfulness in Clinical Practice*. New York: Guilford Press. pp. 205–20.

Loesser, F.H. (1951) 'The Inch Worm', song.

Morgan, A. (undated) An Introduction to Narrative Therapy: The Story of Sean. Available at: www.dulwichcentre.com.au/what-is-narrative-therapy.html

Reid, H.L. and Westergaard, J. (2011) *Effective Counselling with Young People*. Exeter: Learning Matters.

Tolan, J. (2012) *Skills in Person-centred Counselling*. London: Sage.

Twigg, E., Barkham, M., Bewick, B.M., Mulhern, B., Connell, J. and Cooper, M. (2009) 'The young person's CORE: development of a brief outcome measure for young people', *Counselling and Psychotherapy Research*, 9(3): 160–8.

3

DEEPENING AND DEVELOPING COUNSELLING SKILLS

INTRODUCTION

This chapter will explore the counselling skills that are useful for best practice in counselling children and young people. Case studies and activities illustrate how to deepen the counselling relationship through connection with and understanding of our young clients.

Essential counselling skills with children and young people can be broken down into the following elements:

- skills in relating:
  - differences from counselling adults
  - communication styles specific to young clients
- core elements of counselling skills:
  - presence: the skill of being the person you are
  - connection: deepening contact
  - respect: 'I will if you will!'
- developing the relationship:
  - getting below the surface
  - managing diversity issues
  - understanding the 'warp' in the counselling 'mirror': who do you remind me of?
  - going with resistance: 'I don't want to be here and who are you anyway?'
  - allowing quietness
  - accepting endings and moving on.

SKILLS IN RELATING

Differences from counselling adults

The focus of this chapter is on the heart of the matter: the skilful counselling relationship with a young client. We need to learn and practise the distinct counselling skills which apply specifically to children and young people.

Safety, confidentiality, disclosure and protection issues that matter greatly when counselling children and young people will be addressed in later chapters.

Being respectful when with young clients is given particular attention as negative judgement of children is often acceptable in our society and is a 'cultural norm'.

Counsellors may need to modify a parental approach, however subtle and nurturing it may be, and learn to be 'alongside' the young in their journey through counselling. Counselling the young, whether they are 5 or 15, can lead to a sense of being in an unfamiliar land, of not knowing what to do as learnt rules and norms concerning how to best listen, connect and respond do not directly apply.

Some counsellors may find they are more comfortable with child/adolescent styles of communication than they are with counselling adults, whilst others will be more at ease with adults. It is simply useful to remember that child/adolescent counselling is not the same as adult counselling. Skills need to be adapted and modified with new ways of working added.

The therapeutic alliance was identified in Chapter 1 as key to counselling young clients. Here, qualities within that alliance and the skills that need to be applied to make the counselling relationship function well are explained.

Using the skills that work best when counselling children and young people may mean 'unlearning' methods that have been successfully practised with adults. The trained practitioner may attempt to counsel young clients in ways that have been designed for practice with adults who are in later life stages and therefore have differing needs. Some counselling skills apply to all clients and can be directly applicable, whilst other skills are clearly different from those used in counselling adults. There are differences based on the age and developmental stage of the client.

Communication styles specific to young clients

To illustrate the communication style and response needed, consider this:

> A new counselling service based in a hospital was experiencing difficulties in communication with child and adolescent patients in a unit for cancer care. Young clients were, in general, quiet and withdrawn, due, understandably, to their illness and to the sense of being in a strange and 'alien' environment. It was discovered that a change in communication *style* was needed, taking a more active, engaged and less formal approach whilst listening and responding.

> Asking some direct questions, using humour in a careful way and sometimes talking together about something completely different, like football, dance classes, exams or favourite music were strategies that helped. The young patients were able to relax a little and respond rather than feeling 'frozen' in the strange and frightening world of hospital cancer treatment.

As counsellors, there can be an expectation that we will 'just know' how to translate our communication style to children and young people.

The above example shows that there are new skills to develop and great rewards to be found in getting communication with young clients 'right'. For the young, having someone in their lives who is not parent, teacher or other 'authority' figure, and yet has an ethical and insightful approach, is of great value.

CORE ELEMENTS OF COUNSELLING SKILLS

Presence: the skill of being the person you are

We often use phrases like 'bringing ourselves' to the counselling relationship, 'being the self we truly are' and 'walking in the talk' as ways to describe the skill of being congruent in the counselling relationship with young clients. Many adults, particularly if they are already parents or teachers, will put themselves in a 'role' with young clients and offer good, safe techniques that can help. Worksheets that explain what emotions like anger or grief are and ways to 'manage' better can be helpful in a limited way. They do not, however, offer the same level of change as being present with a young client, feeling their suffering and entering into a moment of connection with them. We are in a position to 'walk alongside' young clients in their predicament, whatever it may be.

To offer presence in this way requires courage and the ability to be vulnerable whilst remaining ever the professional counsellor.

Skills for presence:

- being 'here and now'
- giving attention to anything that might obstruct your presence
- mindful noticing
- deep, attentive listening in the present moment.

Being 'here and now' Over many years of counselling young clients, I have been asked by others how the therapeutic relationship is created with a resistant teenager or with a shy, scared child. I previously thought that to create a relationship in counselling, an ability to remember what it was like to be that age and be 'in their shoes' was the key issue. This is part of the answer, but now, as supervisor of many counsellors who have young clients, I find it is presence, bringing yourself into relationship with the client in the 'here and now', that is the essential skill that is pivotal for other skills that will be identified. Green (2010) offers the insight that we need to connect with our heart as well as our head.

Each young client is different from the next, completely unique and individual. Nevertheless, there are features of youth that offer us the opportunity to consider how best to relate to them.

The young can be very open and often have powerful 'bullshit' detectors. If you try to be 'professional' and 'expert' and give any over-simplified solutions, then many youngsters will quickly switch off. An example of this is a glib phrase such as 'you have a choice how you behave and actions have consequences'. Whilst this may be true on one level, such a response, especially near the beginning when the relationship is being formed, is an immediate 'switch off' for most young people. To deny the pain, suffering and confusion in a young client's life that has contributed to and often caused their challenging behaviour is to over-simplify and miss the point. Accepting what the client says and holding respect for them as a person can be a very unusual experience in their young lives.

Our job as counsellors is not to condone or encourage 'bad' or unhelpful behaviour and there will be a time in counselling where action needs to be taken to enable change when the client is ready to do so.

In counselling, young clients have the chance to just be themselves: tired, happy, bored, rude, disinterested or very engaged and attached. They have the space to say 'I want to leave now' after 10 minutes or 'Can we talk about something else?' or 'I wish you had been here yesterday 'cos I am OK today' or 'Please don't tell anyone about what my mum/dad/grandparent/uncle/aunt/carer is doing to me; you are the only person I can trust'.

The essential skill that is needed is for you to be genuinely present with them in counselling. This does not mean disclosing a personal event in your life or becoming over-involved in the client's emotions. You cannot agree to overstep the limits to confidentiality, you don't have to accept rudeness or aggression that is aimed toward you, and you need to know how to manage the attachments that children and young people may form to you as the person who has time to listen to and accept them. It requires high levels of self-awareness and the ability to remain calm to practise presence with young clients in all circumstances.

Giving attention to anything that might obstruct your presence Part of maintaining your presence as a counsellor with children and young people is being honest with yourself. The young are demanding of your presence and are often not as polite as adults have been trained to be. They will often notice the absence behind your eyes when you are not wholly present. On the days when the inevitable 'stuff' in our lives takes over and is in our heart and mind, young clients will suddenly behave in different ways, being perhaps more quiet or more disruptive, depending on their tendencies. We can consider their behaviour, but first let's consider our own psychological 'absence', asking:

- Am I tired, cross or pre-occupied?
- Do I want/need to keep part of my mind elsewhere? With another client, a family member or a friend in need?
- Have I got my own problems that are weighing heavily on me today?
- Am I joyful, full of energy and raring to go?

Most counsellors will remember that they have felt most of the above in their counselling career, but what to do with those feelings? Turning away from these feelings, especially the more negative ones, leaving them 'at home' or 'outside the counselling room' seems to be a way that counsellors are often trained to manage this. Of course, it is necessary to remain in the counsellor 'role'; we need to recognise that it's the client's time not ours. One method of helping to manage strong feelings that preoccupy us is to turn towards them rather than away, not suppressing but shining the light of awareness upon them, giving them some space, making 'friends' with difficulties. This approach helps us access our own inner wisdom (Germer and Seigel 2012).

Just imagine you opened an electricity bill on your way to counselling this morning and it was three times as much as you expected. No time to phone the company – just got to get on with it! Counsellors are trained to put themselves 'aside' and be present for the client – this is the ideal solution but sometimes challenging in practice. Perhaps you are trying to find five minutes in your counselling day to sort out the bill, but it is playing on your mind. Your presence with your client is only partial and your threshold for becoming stressed or grumpy is low.

REFLECTIVE ACTIVITY: STRATEGIES FOR MAINTAINING PRESENCE WHEN HAVING A DIFFICULT DAY

- Turn towards the problem rather than away from it.
- Make notes about how you are feeling.
- Plan a definite time in the day when you will make sure you are able to begin addressing any personal issue that is pre-occupying you.
- Put aside attention to clients during planned breaks.
- Attend to your own needs for food, exercise, fresh air or quietness.
- Make contact with adults, even if it's just a simple greeting during the day.

This links what was begun in Chapter 1 when we considered preparing for the counselling journey. Here, we are deepening the relationship by learning to be more present and attentive.

> ## MINDFUL MOMENT: PRESENCE
>
> Stop what you doing and notice what is happening in your mind and body right now.
>
> - What are your current thoughts?
> - Take some even breaths in and out.
> - Notice what you are thinking of right now.
> - Do your thoughts concern the past, the future or the present?
> - Bring your attention to your feelings – whatever you are feeling is worth noting.
> - Don't try to change your feelings right now – simply bring your full attention to them.
> - Next, notice your bodily sensations.
> - Note whether you are warm or cold, comfortable or uncomfortable.
> - Take a few minutes to consider what helps you to become calm yet alert.
>
> This activity helps to bring you into the present, where you can respond more fully to what is happening right now.

Mindful noticing The skill of mindful noticing with children and young people requires that the counsellor think, feel and connect in the relationship. Knowing what it is like to be the client is so important and yet it is not enough if making that connection causes an emotional reaction that debilitates the counsellor. We are in the privileged position of being witness to both the joys and hardships experienced by young people. This can be painful, frightening and angry-making as well as fun, interesting and surprising. What mindful noticing offers is the ability to be fully with the client. This relies on maintaining calmness whilst knowing both ourselves and the other person. To do this requires commitment to a regular personal practice of self-awareness.

The lives of young clients involve both great suffering and wonderful happiness. Listening to disclosures of loss and pain, as well as being alongside in moments of success, are daily tasks of counsellors whose clients are children and young people.

Deep, attentive listening and responding in the present moment Practise noticing and listening to your inner voice in the present moment. Before you begin, take a moment to stop and do nothing. When counselling, offer this same level of attention to your client (Nhat Hanh 2011).

Connection: deepening contact

- Be on the client's level. This may involve physically sitting on the floor, on a cushion or on a similar chair to the young client's. Teachers often have a bigger chair for practical reasons, but also to symbolise their role, the sense of being 'in authority' and psychologically holding a sense of inequality.

- Recognise that the client knows their own life best and that even very young clients have clear insights into their own situation. A counsellor can never be fully equal with a young client as the roles of counsellor and client are different by nature. A determination to understand life from the 'other' point of view is, however, helped by being on the same level.

- Be yourself and don't try to be the same as the client! This may sound obvious and even strange, but when it comes to teenagers there is often a great need in them to be different; the counsellor not quite understanding, or allowing them to be the expert in, the worlds of technology, film, fashion, music or sport can be very appealing to teens.

- Be aware that younger children tend to learn through imitation and may want to copy the behaviour of their counsellor or idolise them and imagine what it would be like if their counsellor was their parent. It is important for you to recognise how the client sees you and discuss this with your supervisor. (This will be explained in more detail later in the chapter.) How you respond when your client tells you about their life is crucial. You need to discriminate between holding personal opinions and views and challenging dangerous or risky behaviour in your client when you really need to. You may not like something your client does in their life but as long as they are not at risk of significant harm it may be useful to stretch your ability to empathise to include things you have never experienced or thought of before.

- Remember that there will be areas where the young client really does know more than you. Not trying to compete, criticise or even congratulate but rather holding an open and genuine interest in the client's area of knowledge can really facilitate the growth of trust and relational connection between you.

CASE EXAMPLE: JUDE LEARNS TO BOX

You have been counselling Jude for several weeks. She has come to rely on you for emotional support whilst she has been coming to terms with the divorce of her parents and the animosity between them as they refuse to speak to each other. Her older brother has recently left home to join the army. Jude's family are proud of her brother who will soon go overseas. Jude watched young women boxing on television during the Olympics and was impressed. Her PE teacher suggested that she learn to box and now she goes regularly to a club and is starting to compete at local level. As her counsellor, you hold personal opinions about long-term safety issues and the aggressive nature of the sport. You 'try' to show enthusiasm for Jude's new interest but this is challenging your ability to connect with her as you strongly disapprove of her choice of sport.

Dilemma: How do you approach this with Jude when she asks you directly what you think about her boxing?

One way to approach this dilemma is to bring in skills from Transactional Analysis.

Skills from Transactional Analysis (TA)

The practice of TA offers an immediate way to make contact and connect with aspects of a young client. The TA approach offers the idea that different aspects of ourselves will communicate better with different aspects of others. TA considers that we all have an inner parent, adult and child known as 'ego states'. Broadly, the parent deals in shoulds and oughts, caring for others and having ideas and opinions. The inner adult is involved in co-operating, problem solving and thinking. The child holds feelings and the ability to play, be spontaneous and adapt to what others require of us (Fowlie and Sills 2011).

The caring 'parental' response to a direct question

There may be an honest response from the counsellor's 'inner parent'. If this comes from the 'nurturing', caring parent then it could take the form of expressing concern: 'I feel concerned that you might get hurt and that there could be long-term consequences if you get hit on the head often whilst boxing.' This response, if offered thoughtfully and with respect, could give Jude the opportunity to feel cared for and not feel that she is doing something that may risk losing her good connection with you if she wants to continue boxing.

Speaking to the 'emerging adult'

A useful alternative would be to approach this dilemma in an 'adult' manner. The adult approach in TA offers the opportunity for co-operative problem solving and the possibility of both of you offering information to the other. Your response from an 'adult' perspective could be: 'I don't know much about the latest developments in women's boxing, could you tell me more? I think they have improved safety with helmets, is that the case?' This response gives Jude the chance to explain what she knows about her new interest and possibly question some aspects of it she hasn't thought of before.

Joining with the adolescent

A third way to approach answering Jude's question would be to engage your 'inner adolescent', as identified by Geldard and Geldard (2010). Geldard and Geldard extend the TA model of the inner 'parent', 'adult' and 'child' responses to include the response of the inner 'adolescent': 'Oh, boxing, well, that's a surprise, wow, didn't know you'd be up for something like that! Sounds scary too … what do you do? Do you actually fight? Does it hurt?'

This third way offers Jude a way to express her own concerns without sensing that you might judge her. It also offers you, as the counsellor, a chance to express your concerns in a 'lighter' way.

A less useful response to Jude's question

It will depend on the kind of person you are which one of the above options, using TA, would work best for you. What would be less likely to deepen or develop the connection between you and Jude is a response such as:

'Well, I don't know anything about boxing, so I don't really have an opinion; it's not important what I think anyway.'

Many adolescents dislike this kind of response in counselling because they sense it is 'masked' or 'guarded' and can cause an atmosphere of unease. Jude may make a mental note not to talk about boxing again.

Each of us will respond slightly differently when we are in a situation where we hold a strong opinion about a client's behaviour. This is appropriate as we are individuals and the nature of counselling is that we respect individuality, including our own. A counsellor who has had problems with their own eating, for example, may respond differently when a client talks of their 'binges' to a counsellor who has never come across this before.

Responses are more skilful if the relevant personal experiences of the counsellor have been examined and resolved and less skilful if it is a difficult, unresolved subject for the counsellor.

In order to deepen the connection with young clients, it would be useful to make a note of what might be difficult subjects or vulnerable areas for you: areas that you might want to draw away from or be more comfortable not going deeply into. Also make a note of areas you feel you would be comfortable with and confident to explore or discuss in depth.

REFLECTIVE ACTIVITY

For each one of the issues below, write:

- 'C' if you are confident in deeply connecting with that issue if a client brought it to counselling
- 'N' for need to know more, research or find local resources
- 'V' if you find there is a personal vulnerability with this particular issue as it is connected with your own life experience.

Common issues that you will meet in counselling include:

- abuse – physical
- abuse – mental and emotional
- abuse – sexual
- bereavement
- eating disorders/problems

(Continued)

(Continued)

- alcohol – client using
- alcohol – adults in the client's life with alcohol 'problems'
- drugs – illegal
- drugs – prescription
- extreme sports, e.g. free running
- graffiti
- self-harm
- social networking
- computer games with war-like content.

How did you respond to these issues? Remember that your own life experience is often an asset. If you need to know more or feel vulnerable in a particular area, decide on an action you will take to gain the support and information you need.

Counsellors can have strong opinions, e.g. 'it's too much computer time that causes problems'. Such opinions, if unexamined, hinder counselling with the young, for most of whom computers are an integral part of their everyday lives.

As a supervisor, I sometimes learn from supervisees who are very different from me. I may have a more accepting, less solution-focused style than a supervisee who has a background in the NHS, social work or the police, but by listening carefully to their approach and their reasons for their way of counselling I may discover something about myself and modify my views. As counsellors, it is crucial to be open-minded to aspects of young clients' lives that may be unfamiliar to us.

We all make choices and assumptions based on our own experience and training. The importance of discussing and challenging our own opinions and expectations of young clients in order to connect with them cannot be over-emphasised, particularly as young clients are accustomed to being 'told' what to do.

Respect: 'I will if you will!'

Many children and young people have a keen sense of injustice when it comes to respect, feeling they are 'made' to respect others whilst not being respected themselves. Counsellors are good at respecting their young clients, but in some cases this is more difficult, especially if you believe your client is 'making it up' in counselling.

Creative imagination, fibs, fantasy, lies and tall stories

Here are two case studies where the young client brings a story to counselling that is not 'true'. Not telling the truth in counselling can be a symptom of a deep, underlying and possibly unconscious problem. For younger children, making up stories can be fun, a blurring of fact and fantasy or a method of self-protection that has worked well for them in their young lives.

Recognising these possible reasons for 'untruths' does not necessarily make it any easier for the counsellor to manage this situation.

Adults are often highly judgemental of children and young people who lie. The immediate response from some children on being caught for a misdemeanour is 'It wasn't me'! Whilst this can be seen as humorous, in other cases lies are taken very seriously by adults, with punishments being severe.

How can counsellors respond when a young client brings a story about their life that subsequently turns out not to be the 'truth'?

Can the counsellor hold a non-judgemental position and respect their client whilst questioning the veracity of the story they are telling in counselling?

CASE EXAMPLE: MELANIE'S TWIN SISTER

Melanie, aged 8, is brought to see you by her mother. You begin by bringing 'Mum' into the counselling room and explaining how confidentiality will work. You will be discussing anything that means Melanie is at risk with her, but all other topics will be confidential. As Melanie is 8, you will need to talk with her mum about transport and payment and give a general progress report like 'it's going well', or conversely if you assess that Melanie is not benefiting from counselling then you may need to explain to her mother what kind of interventions are preferable.

Melanie has been sexually abused by an uncle. Her younger sister Anna, aged 6, made the disclosure by fleeing to a neighbour's home when the uncle was 'babysitting'. It is clear that Melanie has also been a victim of abuse and confirmed this to her mother when asked, but other than that she has never spoken about her experiences of abuse. All steps have been taken to remove the uncle and the authorities have been informed. One concern of Melanie's mother is that if Melanie is asked to speak about the abuse she will not do so. Melanie's mother has also told you on the phone previously that she is concerned that Melanie plays alone in school, has trouble making friends and tells lies. She is mostly 'good' and 'quiet' – the problems only arise if she is questioned and then she makes up 'stories'. There are odd moments of her scaring her younger sister, Anna, with ghost tales.

Aware of the impact of these circumstances and the possibility of the trial of Melanie's uncle, you plan to focus on listening to, responding to and playing together with Melanie.

Melanie responds very well to the sessions in that she is relaxed and engaged and interacts freely with you. During session three, she tells you all about her twin sister, Monica, who is very mean to their younger sister, Anna. Monica, you

(Continued)

(Continued)

are told, is not kind and helpful at home and scares Anna with ghost stories, steals change that's left around the house and hides Anna's toys and sometimes even breaks them. At first, you feel surprised that Melanie's mother has not mentioned this twin sister. Perhaps Melanie is being blamed for the twin's behaviour.

You are confused and take the issue to supervision. Your supervisor, on hearing the story, asks straightaway if twin sister Monica actually exists, or is it a way of Melanie externalising 'bad' or troubling aspects of her life? You feel caught out when the truth dawns – why didn't you think of that?

Your supervisor encourages you to check out with Melanie's mother how many children are in the family. You do so and it is confirmed that there are two: Melanie and Anna.

So, how do you approach this in counselling, if at all? Next time you meet Melanie, you could say that you have just found out she doesn't have a twin sister and ask her why she told you that she did. What are the advantages and disadvantages of challenging her in this way?

First, consider the case of Jacob, outlined below, and then ask what is involved in deciding how to respond to the child or young person who is 'making it up'.

CASE EXAMPLE: JACOB'S MARTIAL ARTS

Jacob is 16 when he comes to see you. He has been referred by a tutor who has described him as withdrawn. Jacob tells you about his love of martial arts and how he plans to go and train with monks in China to further his abilities. As his counsellor, you are exploring and learning more about him. You ask a couple of questions about where he goes to classes and what particular style of martial arts he practises. After a while, you begin to feel confused by his responses. You decide not to question him further as you had only been focusing on the martial arts as a way to build the therapeutic alliance. Jacob doesn't want to talk about any relationships in his life and after an opening conversation about his week, he returns to the topic of martial arts and speaks in a distant way about going to China and gaining black-belt status. As you listen, there is a growing sense of Jacob's world being one of fantasy, a world that is taking place in virtual reality, in his room at home via his laptop. Jacob does not ever say that he is imagining himself as a great martial artist, but you begin to sense that he has never been to an actual martial arts lesson.

You take the issue to supervision as you feel torn between just listening and being interested in his story and wanting to reflect back some inconsistencies in what he is saying and tell him of the growing discomfort you feel, holding an

> awareness that others around him will also find it difficult to connect with him, thus leading to the isolation and withdrawal that he is experiencing. You also understand that there will be underlying reasons why Jacob finds it safer to be in a world of his own. During discussions with your supervisor, you find a real sense of dilemma between being open, expressing your discomfort with the story around his martial arts practice and then challenging him to be more open with you or simply allowing him to talk, to 'suspend disbelief' and give him respect for his version of reality that may have been in short supply in his life until now.

These case studies are designed to challenge our ability to respect a young client unconditionally. Can we say I will accept you, but not your story if it is not true?

Counsellors will meet the situation of clients withholding, lying, manipulating 'truth' or holding incorrect negative beliefs about themselves, others or their world. The extensive fantasy lives of the young may be part of coping with difficult life circumstances and need to be understood and dealt with sensitively and carefully.

When discussing counselling adolescents, Geldard and Geldard (2010: 89) say:

> We will listen to the young person's story and will accept it at face value as the young person's truth even if the story stretches our credulity. We will be totally accepting of the story and will not challenge its veracity.

They go on to explain that often young people have stories to tell that are difficult to believe and may be true. Geldard and Geldard (2010) say they know some counsellors will disagree with the suggestion that we should always believe the client, but they explain that clients are likely to re-evaluate their 'constructs' and come nearer to objective truth as trust develops.

A very helpful example of how to counsel a client who is lying is offered by Brice, who offers the story of a young adult man who lies about many things, including his mother's death. Brice writes about his own response to this: 'I felt angry at being deceived. I felt stupid, a fraud and really challenged about my worth as a counsellor' (cited in Tolan 2012: 80).

Within the counselling, Brice and his client learned to trust the relationship and were able to make jokes about 'making it all up' after the truth was revealed by chance. This offered both counsellor and client an opportunity to learn and grow. Brice was left with the knowledge that he could accept a client and their lying 'without rancour, without regret for me and with as much positive regard for them as I can find' (cited in Tolan 2012: 82).

These examples offer the opportunity for us to learn how to be fully present with the child or young person, whatever 'story' they are telling us.

I remember being shocked when a casual remark from a youth worker helped me to understand that a client had been telling me a story that wasn't true. As with Brice, there were feelings of being foolish, and a wave of anger and rejection followed. Perhaps the young client was 'wasting my time' or not 'using the counselling properly'.

Counsellors can be encouraged to be judgemental by parents, teachers, etc. who do not like the idea of accepting a young person who is telling 'made-up stories'. If we do decide as counsellors to accept a young client's story when it may not be true, we need to know the basis on which we are doing so. Brice asks in his conclusion if we counsellors may present only a partial truth of ourselves to the client – a falseness that may encourage the lie.

Certainly, a bitter complaint from some young people towards adults who judge them is that the adult is not offering mutuality or respect: *'Adults want us to be polite, but they are not polite to us.'* This seems to be an acceptable way of behaving for many adults, so the unconditional acceptance being explained here will be a very different view from that of other adults in the young person's experience.

When, however, the possibility of significant harm arises, safety concerns will need to be considered. When the young client is at possible risk of harm to themselves or others, then you must consider whether the 'untruth' is too risky to accept.

Challenging a client's story takes skill and it is important to get the timing right and hold the client's best interests firmly as the most important consideration, not being influenced by what teachers or parents might think as to when and how the story is challenged. Always keep the acceptance and respect of the client as a person at the heart of any challenging intervention, not allowing any sense of being 'caught out' by believing a 'lie' to influence you.

Do's and don'ts when challenging the young client's story

Do:

- make it clear that you accept your client wholly as the young person they are and, if their story turns out to be untrue, it will not affect their entitlement to counselling

- consult with your supervisor and discuss whether challenging the story is the best available choice

- find the best moment to challenge; you can always return to a subject with your client in a later session, saying you remember something they said in the past and want to explore it further

- be specific and adopt a tentative, curious approach, saying exactly what you have noticed that doesn't fit for you and wondering how what they have told you is possible

- use the challenge itself as an opportunity to deepen connection, framing your words very positively as a way to gain trust, e.g. 'Most things we talk about make sense to me, but this puzzles me and I can't quite understand how that can be what happened. Can we explore it a bit more?'

- remember that truth can be stranger than fiction. Odd, frightening and horrific stories may, unfortunately, be completely true, so do keep an open mind and hesitate before drawing the conclusion that a story is untrue.

Don't:

- use challenge to question, dismiss or disbelieve a young client on the grounds that you feel uncomfortable or doubtful about a disclosure of abuse or neglect. Children may have been disbelieved in the past and it is crucial that counsellors accept the disclosure and act appropriately (see Chapter 5)

- use 'should' or 'shouldn't', 'ought' or 'must' when challenging. It is never an inquisition!

- challenge because another person (teacher, parent, etc.) says they want to know about something in the child or young person's life and tells you what they want you to ask

- make fun of or joke about something a client has said to challenge a story. However 'jokey' the sessions are, challenges need to be calm and considered.

When you think a disclosure of confidential information is needed, it is necessary to consult with either your clinical supervisor or a trusted experienced peer. Ensure there is no leaking of information until you are clear that disclosure will be in the best interests of the child or young person. Your client has trusted you with their most difficult and hidden personal story and you must honour that trust by making careful and considered disclosures when absolutely necessary. This does not mean waiting, as delays may not be best for the client if they are in some kind of danger or if other children could be in danger from an adult the client has been harmed by in the past. (See Chapter 5 where in-depth information will be offered on confidentiality and professional issues.)

Examples of when you need to consult your supervisor and consider disclosure include:

- A girl (aged 12) who tells you she is eating regularly whilst losing weight dramatically each week and becoming visibly unwell. Friends and family have expressed concerns to you but currently no action is being taken as everyone is hoping this is just a 'phase'.

- An 11-year-old boy who tells you he never drinks alcohol whilst smelling strongly of it during counselling sessions and having lots of problems with managing school, family and friendship groups. He says he is fine and doesn't really want to continue with counselling.

- A 9-year-old boy who repeatedly tells you that marks on his body are from falls when they clearly look like signs of having been beaten. The boy is very jumpy and appears both afraid and over-alert.

- A 17-year-old who discloses she was sexually abused over a number of years by her step-father. She has now moved out of home and is living with her friend's family. She thinks it was just her that her step-father picked on and believes her younger half-brothers and sisters, aged 9, 7 and 3, who are the biological children of her step-father and her mother, are safe at home.

- A 5-year-old who, during play with a toy car, whisperingly tells you how her father picked her up by the neck and shook her when she played with the car at home. She graphically acts out this event on a doll in the therapy room. She says she couldn't breathe and was very scared. She says daddy can be nice sometimes.

- A 14-year-old girl who talks with you about the new boyfriend whom she has met online, who she thinks is 17. It's good fun, she says, and the other day he asked her to show him her breasts online. She says she lifted up her t-shirt for the webcam, but kept her bra on 'this time'. She is looking forward to her next virtual 'meeting' with him.

Unlike the two case studies of Melanie and Jacob, risks are present in these cases and you need to consult with others who 'need to know' and choose the best course of action. This does bring a limitation to the unconditional acceptance counsellors can offer.

There is the possibility of unintended and unknown consequences when the client is young and still developing their own capacity to recognise when they are in danger. Balancing the need to believe and accept stories with risk factors that are not understood by the client is an important consideration.

Where no such risks are evident, and this is in the majority of cases, it is best to accept the client's story unconditionally, however unlikely the tale is, and, with a focus on building the therapeutic alliance, gain enough trust so that clients feel able to share more of themselves.

Respect can be nurtured by remembering that children and young people are just like us. It can be useful to say to yourself: s/he tells lies 'just like me', has problems in their family 'just like me', wants to be or do better 'just like me'. This aspect of respecting, joining with or remembering being young is helped by the following activity.

REFLECTIVE ACTIVITY: JUST LIKE ME/ DIFFERENT FROM ME

Now is the time to remember your own childhood and what it was like to be young. If you have your own children at home and their friends visit, take a new, fresh view of your children and what works and doesn't work when communicating with them.

Alternatively, go out and meet children and young people, through friends, clubs and volunteering.

The most useful counselling skills with children and young people will be based on your ability to be present and congruent with the young. This is both a challenging and rewarding task, and not always an easy one, as often there are judgements and fears, the desire to 'get it right' and expectations – both those of the counsellor and those of parents, teachers, employers and young clients themselves – which get in the way.

All of us will have some pre-conceptions and judgements – even the judgement that young people are 'great' does not take into account the diversity of the young.

The counsellor's own background, their reasons for becoming a counsellor with children and young people, is relevant too. It is not important *what* the background is, rather it's about understanding how that motivation and history make the counsellor who they are.

To start with ourselves, we need to understand the type of young person's counsellor we are and why we want to counsel or are counselling children and young people.

REFLECTIVE ACTIVITY: YOUR CHILDHOOD AND ADOLESCENCE

If possible, sit in a room where you counsel or, alternatively, sit in a quiet place where you will be uninterrupted.

Sit in the counsellor's chair and imagine yourself as a 7-year-old sitting in the client's chair. Take time to look, sense and feel what your 7-year-old self is like. What is your 7-year-old self wearing? Is s/he comfortable in the 'client's' chair? Take time to gather as much information as you can and, when you are ready, change places and become the 7-year-old you, looking at the counsellor 'you'. What does the 7-year-old you say/do/feel/think?

Take time to discover as much as possible and then, when you are ready, return to the 'counsellor' seat. Thank your 7-year-old self and say 'farewell' to them, returning to the present where you are alone in your counselling room or quiet place.

Write notes about what happened in this encounter. Remember that there are no 'right' and 'wrong' ways that this type of exercise can develop. You may choose to gain support from your supervisor or a colleague to discuss the exercise. If you cannot contact your 7-year-old self, this is worth noting, in a non-judgemental way.

Repeat the exercise, after a gap for processing, to meet with your 11-year-old, 14-year-old and 18-year-old selves. There will be differences in meeting with each age. When you meet, in the exercise, with your teenage 'selves', there will be more opportunity for questioning, Pay attention to how each of the various ages views you as the counsellor. Noting down your responses will give you an opportunity to become familiar with the basis upon which you respond when counselling young clients of various ages.

Give yourself plenty of time to complete this exercise and then consider what you have discovered.

In my own experience, the 7-year-old ran over and hugged me and thanked me for being there.

The 11-year-old was troubled and confused but was finding her way by learning to be naughty and secretive (necessary skills in her particular circumstances).

The 14-year-old, angry and rebellious, could hardly bear to be in the same room with me and saw me (the counsellor) as 'weird' and 'fuddy duddy'. I particularly enjoy counselling 14-year-olds now, perhaps because I know the discomfort of my 'inner' 14-year-old so well!

The 18-year-old 'me' I met was a beautiful, kind, independent young woman, and meeting her was a poignant, memorable and surprising experience. I had been quite judgemental when thinking about myself at this age.

Everyone who participates in this activity will have a unique experience. Trust whatever you find and share what is relevant or helpful with your supervisor, a friend or colleague.

DEVELOPING THE RELATIONSHIP

Recently, a trainee counsellor spoke very passionately to me about the feeling of being 'deskilled' – not knowing what to do when a client is a vulnerable young person.

Many adults have lost (or mislaid) the ability to just be with young people. It may be a long time since you were given homework, told what you must wear or what time to go to bed. It may also be ages since you just played with your friends for a whole afternoon in the garden, watched cartoons or hung out all Saturday afternoon in your local town. Remembering that these are the common experiences of your client group will help you to counsel them.

Getting below the surface

REFLECTIVE ACTIVITY: THE FIRST IMPRESSION

Find approximately 10 pictures of children and young people. If possible, make them varied and not caricatures. Make sure they are not known to you or others who you may show them to. Choose different dress styles, age groups, ethnic origins, gender, class, social groups, etc.

Study the pictures yourself and note your initial responses. Do you have strong likes and dislikes? Can you identify any personal prejudices? If you don't like, for example, baseball caps worn backwards, jeans that are torn or shocking pink frilly dresses, it's best to be *aware* of this.

Do you make assumptions based on how a child or young person looks? You may immediately think you don't, but sometimes these assumptions are subtle and based on our own early experiences.

Try the pictures you have found with other adults, partners, friends or colleagues, noting their first responses.

Counsellors can be unable to recognise their own biases and assumptions because they are such strong advocates for children and young people.

Perhaps assumptions and judgements counsellors make are more often about the parents and teachers of children they counsel? For example, if a child looks unkempt, is there an immediate urge to want to protect this child from the 'neglectful' parent who has allowed them to be like this?

Managing diversity issues

There are some very obvious differences between counsellor and client when the client group consists of children and young people. It is simplistic to say that one difference is age, but the importance of remembering what this age difference means in practice cannot be overlooked.

Counsellors have the potential to be powerful and even manipulative. There is a tendency for counsellors to forget that their young clients may not understand what counselling is because of a lack of life experience. Is counselling just a word that we are so familiar with that we assume others understand it?

It is unlikely that young children will have much idea what counselling means. There is a real responsibility, if we are the first counsellor in that child or young person's life, to show, model and explain what counselling is. A different kind of explanation from one that would be given to an adult is required. Often, the words 'you don't have to come to counselling if you don't want to' come as a surprise and are met with quizzical looks from younger children. Some children don't get many choices offered to them. The age difference between us and our clients means our right to make our own life choices differs greatly from theirs.

We may also find differences in religious and moral values, style, culture and language.

Religious and moral values

Knowing that we have different religious beliefs from our young client, we may need to ask them about how growing up in their religion influences their life choices. Showing that we accept a religious style of dress or a need to be absent on particular holy days is vital to developing the counselling relationship.

Style

How do we respond to particular clothes, piercings, tattoos, unusual hair colours and styles? These aspects of young people's lives are so important to them that our response to them can make or break a counselling relationship.

Culture

How much do 'ethnocentric' beliefs influence our counselling of young clients? Do we expect children and young people to 'fit in' to the context we counsel them in or expect them to be like us?

Language

How do you approach counselling the client whose first language is not the same as yours? What is your opinion on swearing?

Gaining insight about your beliefs and concepts, rather than presuming that we are all the same, will help to gain trust and decrease the chance that we will take on the 'expert', 'teacher' or 'parental' role when we are counselling. This does not mean that we exclude adult knowledge or wisdom that may come with age; it simply means that we increase openness and recognise, question and modify any opinions that are not useful to our clients or to us as counsellors.

Understanding the 'warp' in the counselling 'mirror'

Whatever the counselling or therapy orientation you are trained in (see Chapter 4), it is useful to consider the way that a young client sees you when they enter the counselling room and how you may respond to this view of you. In another context, you may have a different view or opinion of them and they will view you differently. I notice that I am pretty much invisible to lots of youngsters. The way that I play, especially computer games, is a surprise to them; I am often ignored with my greying hair and middle-aged appearance!

If the same youngster came into my counselling room, a very different connection would be made. I would immediately make contact with them, saying my name and welcoming them to counselling. In many cases, rapport will have been established within the first few minutes and we might be smiling at each other or seriously talking about what has brought them to counselling. The contact is entirely different from meeting the same youngster in a social situation.

The effect of this difference is profound: as counsellors, we are skilled in forming a bond for the purposes of allowing the client to feel safe enough to open up about their private life. In doing so, we can create a 'warp'.

The counsellor is seen, often, as more than an ordinary human person. The warmth and open-heartedness in the contact that is offered can give rise to being seen as rather wonderful or even terrifying by young clients. This asks of counsellors of the young that they be responsible to a very high standard and respect the strength of feeling that may be created as a result of forming this relationship.

CASE EXAMPLE: THE INVISIBLE CHILD

A young girl comes to counselling who is the fifth out of six children. She is experiencing some bullying at school and is often found crying in the playground. The school feels she needs some support. Her parents know she is coming to counselling but are concerned that she isn't over-protected; their view is that she needs to toughen up a bit. When she meets you, she is very shy and withdrawn. After a while, she begins to 'come out of her shell' and enjoys talking, laughing, playing and expressing her struggles with you. She never misses a session and expresses surprise when you say something 'nice' to her. She is 'invisible' in her home life, mainly spoken to when asked to do a job or told to go to bed or 'be quiet'. She doesn't remember being complimented at home, as her siblings are generally better than her at most things.

Suddenly, the light of attention, of care and consideration is on her for one hour a week and she draws it in with every pore in her body. She never sees that you are an ordinary human with your own problems and challenges. To her, you are lovely, kind and accepting and she is happy for the time she is with you, even if she is expressing difficulties with others.

Perhaps you remind clients of someone else or, alternatively, something about their appearance or demeanour means that you have made decisions about them before counselling begins. It is very likely that we will pick up an 'atmosphere' or feel a response to our clients when we are in a therapeutic relationship with them.

Babette Rothschild (1993) gives us a way of understanding this by considering 'mirror neurons'. Mirror neurons suggest that what we pick up from clients is physiological; that as counsellors and therapists, when we enter into relationship, empathise and connect with clients, we are actually adapting ourselves to connect with the client in ways that we may not be aware of.

REFLECTIVE ACTIVITY

Young clients may transfer onto you the image of:

- good parent
- grown-up friend
- confidante
- auntie or uncle
- big sister/brother or other family member
- fairy godmother/father
- witch/wizard
- kind but rather stupid person they can 'control'
- spy for their parents/teacher to find out their secrets.

Choose any that resonate from the list or add your own and just imagine for a moment what your response to being 'seen' in this way might be. What feelings could be generated in you?

Our responses can be unnoticed by us or misunderstood as we are invited into being, for example, the 'rescuing parent' for a child in distress.

The following case study offers an example of how the young client believes something about their counsellor which is not seeing them for who they are, but rather as who they would like their counsellor to be. The counsellor, in turn, responds to this by taking on the role that the young client wishes for in their life.

> ## CASE EXAMPLE: THE MAGICAL WIZARD
>
> Jeremy, aged 6, is referred to a male counsellor when his dad dies. Jeremy's dad had cancer but did not like to talk about it. Jeremy is the youngest of four children and there is a view held by most adults in his life that he doesn't really understand the 'ins and outs' of what has happened and it is best to just be as normal with him as possible. It was decided that Jeremy shouldn't attend the funeral of his father, so a neighbour cared for him on the day which is now about seven months ago. Since then, Jeremy has become withdrawn at school and there is a consensus that he is not 'getting over' the bereavement. During counselling, Jeremy talks about his own private world that is a world of wizards and magic. He sees you, his counsellor, as a magical being who is casting good spells on him. This is his way of understanding the therapeutic process, as it feels like magic to him. In turn, you as his counsellor begin to feel that you are lifting the mist, confusion and sadness that have surrounded him since his dad died. You notice you feel 'magical' when the two of you are together and enjoy creating imaginary cloaks, happiness spells and vanquishing potions that send teachers who shout into invisibility for a while. You recognise that this approach is having a beneficial influence on Jeremy and occasionally have a concern about whether Jeremy really believes you are 'magic'. Sometimes you feel you really have magical powers in sessions with him!

It is easy to think that such a positive transferral both for counsellor and client is not an issue, and some modalities of counselling and therapy will place more emphasis on this than others. Babette Rothschild (1993) offers a 'common-sense approach' with two key qualities:

- **acceptance** – accepting that the nature of counselling relationships and the therapeutic alliance will bring up strong connections or aversions in both client and counsellor. If you take a particularly strong dislike to a young client, feel strongly attached to them or find yourself feeling something that is unusual for you, take this to supervision. The mistake is to believe in it too much. If you find that you are categorising someone a 'horrible child' or 'so lovely I could take them home' or even feeling magical and able to create spells, then take this to supervision and don't think it's 'just how it is'

- **honesty** – this means finding the appropriate way to say what is happening in the counselling, both to the client and to your supervisor. With young clients, what you say to them needs to be age-appropriate. In the case of Jeremy above, you may want to let him know at some point that you are not magic and that he, Jeremy, is making changes with your help. This can be done within a kind, gentle, client-centred framework; there is no question of taking away what has been a very supportive way for him to manage in troubled times.

You could, for example, explain to Jeremy that your 'powers' to make him feel better are really skills you have learnt that he could learn too. Then help him to discover his own inner resources and safe places that are always available to him, rather than existing inside you, his counsellor.

If it is hard for you to let go of the 'role', then this is a sign that something needs to change.

Using immediacy

Speaking about what is happening in the present, in the room right now, can help to resolve any problems that might arise through being seen in a certain way by your client.

When a young client has been abused or neglected and suffered very deeply, a counsellor or therapist may feel overwhelmed by the client's feelings and experiences. The response of wanting to rescue the client can also be very powerful and be troubling and confusing for the counsellor.

How can we 'be' with an innocent child who has been betrayed by the adults who are supposed to care for her/him?

CASE EXAMPLE: MEG'S CHORES

Meg is 14 and has to get up at 5.00 am to do all her chores. If she doesn't finish, she tells you that her family won't take her to the bus stop to get the school transport. If she misses the bus, she has to walk 11 miles to school or stay at home. When you are in the counselling room with Meg, you notice that she flinches a lot – you suspect that she is subjected to a lot of physical punishment, possibly abuse, but Meg has not told you that this is the case. She has said that she is the only child in her family to be treated in this way – somewhere between a servant and a slave to her brothers, step-mother and father. She is not allowed to eat with the family, gets leftovers and then retreats to her room if she can to do her homework. She also tells you that her family regularly tell her she is useless and bad.

Someone from social services has visited the family and been told that Meg is a dramatic girl with a vivid imagination. The house is clean and tidy so social services are satisfied that Meg's home life is acceptable. No one except you has spoken to her in depth. You are particularly concerned by the fear she exudes and the sense of her 'cowering' when challenged. You express concern to your supervisor and to her year head at the school where you counsel. The school often finds a way to feed Meg as she isn't given a packed lunch and often has no money to buy food.

As her counsellor, you begin to feel helpless and victimised yourself, angry with her family and with social services who, you are sure, are missing the signs

(Continued)

> *(Continued)*
>
> of abuse and neglect. You start to feel overwhelmed by sorrow when you know Meg is coming to counselling. You begin to sense you are failing her and talk to your supervisor extensively – perhaps to the extent of not being able to give time to reflect on other clients. You begin to think of her every day, even though you see her once a week and try to think of ways to get social services to review the case again.
>
> Whilst it is important to keep trying to find help for Meg, it is vital to understand how seriously being involved in cases like this can affect you.

Camila Batmanghelidjh, psychotherapist and founder of Kids Company, writes: 'If you ever want to escape this experience (of being overwhelmed), stand still instead to observe the learning. The feelings transferred onto you hold information which can inform your interventions' (2006: 53).

In this case, the feelings of utter loss and inability to cope or change anything may well be Meg's feelings that you are picking up, as she is not fully able to express how life is for her.

Understanding and recognising this is useful and will help you to offer counselling or therapy in a more skilful way. You may also find the way forward to act on Meg's behalf by fully acknowledging what you are experiencing when you counsel her.

Going with resistance: 'I don't want to be here and who are you anyway?'

Remember that it's a characteristic of adolescents to be rebellious and challenge adults. If a client in their teens expresses initial reservations about counselling, welcome any questions or challenges they bring.

- Don't take it personally if a teenager says they don't need counselling, don't like you or don't want to talk about it.
- Try to go with the resistance, perhaps saying that you may have felt the same at their age (if that is true) or that they are wise to not just take counselling at face value – why should they express deep feelings to a stranger? What evidence is there that it will help?
- Consider that humour can work for some counsellors, e.g. 'You are not the first person to think I am weird, my son has often thought so'.
- Explain that counselling should never be compulsory, but ask, why not give it a try just for today?
- Use diversions and card games or ask everyday questions, e.g. about music they like, and show interest whether the answers are to your taste or not. You can say if their

music taste is opposite to yours – creative disagreement can be a fun challenge! Holding the respectful view that the client's choices have equal weight and validity to yours will be a good experience for the young client and will 'model' how their deeper feelings will be treated if they do 'open up' to you later.

Resistance in younger children is different; it may be fear based or simply shyness. Counselling is a very different experience to the everyday lives of most children.

- Use stories or play to reassure and get to know the child (see Chapter 7 on play).
- Consider that it may be appropriate to bring a parent/carer into counselling with a young child and together talk about what is going to happen and what a 'feeling' is, what will happen at the end of the session, how they will be collected and by whom.
- Run shorter sessions if a child seems nervous or unsure in counselling. Take counselling at the child's pace – sometimes just a few minutes of play or a few words spoken will have an effect and are enough for that day.

Allowing quietness

Allowing quietness in the counselling room, even encouraging a moment of keeping still, can be helpful to young clients. Sometimes less is more. Stillness and 'doing nothing' are a rare luxury. This is not the same as teaching relaxation or breathing exercises, as techniques can be over-used. It is better to just allow clients to find their own way to be quiet and still.

> **MINDFUL MOMENT**
>
> Try this for yourself right now.
> Just stop reading and be quiet for a moment. Notice what happens, what fills your mind. Notice everything you can: agitation, relief, boredom or delight.
> Write down your responses and consider how and when you can offer this 'space' to your clients.

Occasionally, long silences develop in counselling with children and young people. It is helpful if we can tolerate and allow this and don't find it necessary to be 'doing' something all the time. Counsellors can feel uncomfortable with silence so practise being quiet and allow the same of young clients.

There are clients who find it very difficult to talk. This is not the same as quietness; rather it is an inability to communicate verbally.

These young clients may want us to take the lead in communication in a way that counsellors can find counter-intuitive. This situation can be found in clients with abuse or neglect in their home environment, where it has been dangerous for them to speak, or with clients who have a condition such as Aspergers or Down's syndrome. In these cases, play or other activities can be the key to building a relationship. (Play strategies will be covered in Chapter 7.)

Accepting endings and moving on

- 'You are the only one who understands and I don't want to stop counselling.'
- 'I am really glad this is the last session. I feel much better now and I can go to my club at this time next week.'
- 'Mum thinks I should be over it by now so I don't think she will be bringing me for much longer.'

These are examples of endings. Sometimes clients just don't turn up anymore; we are in the middle of a therapeutic relationship and they are gone.

You may never know why a client stops coming. You or another adult may ask a client if they want to return to counselling and they may say no, offering no explanation.

This can be very concerning for the counsellor, or there may be relief if a very full caseload means that focusing on those who do want to come and letting go of those who are not engaging, is necessary.

Skills for endings

- Be sure to explain near the beginning of counselling what the time limits are. If you are working in a context that offers short-term counselling, perhaps six sessions, then clients need to know this from the outset.
- Let young clients know as you come near to the last session that the end is approaching, and go over what has been learnt and what has changed.
- Appreciate that sometimes life becomes more difficult for the client during the time they are being counselled. Life may be worse or more problematic than near the beginning of counselling. You may have the option of extending the counselling or offering longer-term counselling.
- Most importantly, be clear with your client what you can and cannot offer them. If you have to stop counselling them, find the best way to end.

ACTIVITY: A WAY OF ENDING

The box of resources: clarifying gains made in counselling

If possible, use an actual box, bag or other container that the young client can keep. Sometimes it is too risky for a young client to take anything home that reveals anything about the counselling. In this case, a 'metaphorical' container can be created, an invisible safe place, where the client can remember the counselling and their relationship with you.

Feeling words, poems, pictures and memories can all be placed in the box. This needs to be framed positively as a safe way to feel stronger, more resourceful and able to cope with whatever life offers.

Imagine what you would put in a box like this – maybe a book, a film, a memory of a place.

If a youngster has been bereaved, it can be useful to put a quality of the person who has died in a resource box rather than just their name. The memory of the person may bring sadness whereas remembering a grandmother's wonderful quality – for example, 'she always called me her little chick and gave me a big hug; I felt safe and loved' – can bring feelings of warmth whilst still acknowledging the loss. Encouraging the idea that a grandmother's love is not lost, but now exists inside and has shown us how to be loving towards others, is an example of the resource or gift that can be found within the darkness of a loss. This type of activity helps to overcome the 'taboos' young people meet against focusing on death (Luxmoore 2012).

Sometimes a young client's ability to cope with the ending of counselling can be very good and it may be harder for the counsellor to end. On other occasions, the counselling has truly been a lifeline for the young client and the ending is very difficult for them.

Make sure you have done all you can to explain to your client how they can get support without you. You may, for example:

◆ give them details of helplines

◆ teach them skills of communication, including how to make feelings and thoughts known and heard safely

◆ ask the client's permission to pass on information to others who may misunderstand their behaviour and might be kinder if they understood more

◆ offer ways to get in contact with you, if that is possible after the counselling ends

◆ hold a review session after a period of time, possibly after two to three months, to talk through how everything is progressing

◆ encourage the idea that everything gained is inside them, not you and explain that they can carry forward gains made long after the counselling is over.

CHAPTER SUMMARY

This chapter has explained some key issues in developing counselling with children and young people. Practising these skills will enable counsellors to engage young clients with more ease, offering ways to develop the relationship:

- Deepen and develop the counselling through awareness of presence, respect and diversity issues.
- Recognise how young people view counsellors and how clients' problems may impact on us.
- Know when is the best time to challenge and when to accept stories that may be 'made up'.
- Offer opportunities for quietness and reflection.
- Give time and attention to endings.

REFERENCES

Batmanghelidjh, C. (2006) *Shattered Lives: Children who Live with Courage and Dignity*. London: Jessica Kingsley.
Fowlie, H. and Sills, C. (eds) (2011) *Relational Transactional Analysis: Principles in Practice*. London: Karnac Books.
Geldard, K. and Geldard, D. (2010) *Counselling Adolescents*. London: Sage.
Germer, C.K. and Seigel, R.D. (eds) (2012) *Wisdom and Compassion in Psychotherapy: Deepening Mindfulness in Clinical Practice*. New York: Guilford Press, p. 30.
Green, J. (2010) *Creating the Therapeutic Relationship in Counselling and Psychotherapy*. Exeter: Learning Matters.
Luxmoore, N. (2012) *Young People: Death and the Unfairness of Everything*. London: Jessica Kingsley.
Nhat Hanh, T. (2011) *Planting Seeds: Practicing Mindfulness with Children*. Berkeley, CA: Parallax Press.
Rothschild, B. (1993) A Common Sense Approach to Transference and Counter Transference. Available at: www.toddlertime.com/mh/terms/countertransference-transference-2.htm
Tolan, J. (2012) *Skills in Person-Centred Counselling*. London: Sage.

4

EXTENDING MODALITIES TO COUNSEL CHILDREN AND YOUNG PEOPLE

INTRODUCTION

This chapter will explore how different modalities in counselling can be modified and extended to fit young clients. Each modality covered includes exercises that are useful to enhance the skills of counselling children and young people. The sections in this chapter are designed to be approached flexibly. If an exercise from any part of this chapter is the right one for your client in your particular circumstances and you are comfortable with it, then use it!

Practise the exercises with colleagues and try them on yourself before using them with clients.

Methods of extending skills are offered for counsellors and therapists whose modality is:

- integrative
- cognitive-behavioural
- psychodynamic
- person-centred and humanistic
- systemic
- narrative.

Particular strengths of each modality for counselling young clients are also identified.

INITIAL TRAINING

All trainings that are designed for counselling adults will give some skills that are relevant for counselling younger clients. These trainings alone are not enough to be competent to counsel children and young people. Even the basic skills of listening and responding need to be modified when counselling the young. (Online resources for developing initial counsellor training to become skilled with children and young people can be found at www.counsellingminded.com)

Consider the differences between listening and attending to a 6-year-old and a 56-year-old. The idea of 'active listening' takes on a whole new shape when a bouncy or shy young child is our client. A 16-year-old offers yet another challenge. Each child, young person and adult we counsel is different and totally individual. We can recognise, though, that there are particular ways that will help us to connect with each age group.

Consider differences in counsellors – they may be the age of the parent or grandparent of the young client and their life experience can be vastly different.

As well as the diversity that needs to be taken into consideration, there are differences in the modality or 'school' of counselling each counsellor has been trained in. Often, training brings about beliefs that this way of counselling is 'right' and another way 'wrong'. For example, when I first witnessed 'motivational interviewing' I thought the counsellor was deliberately doing it 'wrong'. The deep-seated belief that I hold never to 'lead' or make definite suggestions to the client seemed to me to be violated by this approach. Since this time, I have come to understand and appreciate the value of motivational interviewing in some circumstances with young people and find that, practised skilfully, in a client-centred way, it can be very helpful. I particularly like the idea of 'rolling with resistance' rather than opposing resistance (Miller and Rollnick 2002), which is a very good way of interacting with teenagers.

Each modality, every counselling approach, has great strengths. Recognising how a particular approach works with this client group and how best to implement it with any particular client are key to helping the young in counselling.

In my supervision practice, I have found the way that counsellors respond varies depending on the modality of their initial training. Those trained in person-centred counselling may prefer to allow the client to form the agenda rather than being proactive. Those with cognitive-behavioural therapy (CBT) training may want to try and change faulty ways of thinking and behaving in their client rather than consider how their client's home life and past experiences have formed the situation. Those trained in psychodynamic ways may deeply investigate early experiences rather than prioritising being in the 'here and now', offering presence and deep listening.

How we were trained will influence the ways in which we adapt our knowledge and skills to counselling children and young people. The following exercises can be used by all counsellors. They have been divided into sections for counsellors to be able to find ways in which their particular type of training can be adapted and extended.

INTEGRATIVE

Counsellors who have been trained to integrate in their initial training may find many of the exercises given in this chapter of use in the way they are applied to counselling children and young people. It will just depend which modalities have been integrated into an approach to counselling as to how this chapter is used.

The activities offer practical ways to make counselling appropriate for young clients. So the best way to use them is:

- Consider your initial training in counselling.
- What are your strengths? For example, do you know the language of Transactional Analysis (TA) very well or have you never come across this way of counselling before?
- Stay with what you know well as a way of making first contact with your client.
- Relax, listen, respond.
- Begin by forming a therapeutic alliance with your client, and get on their 'wavelength' through empathy, acceptance and presence (see Chapter 3).
- Reflect on the age, life experience and learning abilities of your client.
- Together with your supervisor, if possible, or with your 'inner supervisor' (see Chapter 8), decide on methods that may work best with this particular client. For example, a child whose family has recently changed radically through divorce and re-marriage of their parents will be helped by the 'Stone People' exercise below, in the section for CBT counsellors. A silent, withdrawn child might respond to drawing or a play activity (see Chapter 7).
- Emphasise examining your responses, thoughts and feelings about this client rather than just applying techniques.
- Allow yourself to respond to this particular client and, if this is helpful, use any of the exercises as 'tools' to facilitate the counselling relationship.
- Become familiar with a new exercise before using it with a young client, preferably using it on a training course or as a peer group activity.
- If you try an exercise and it does not go how you imagined it, learn from that. For example, if a child doesn't want to share their 'family tree' (see below) with you, accept that refusal, unlike teachers or parents that might insist on or encourage compliance. Your openness and child-centred approach will offer a new perspective and an opportunity to build trust.

Activity: Using TA to change communication patterns

Some children and young people have learnt words and ways of communicating with adults and each other that are very unhelpful to them. Across the age groups, skills can be learnt by the young that may immediately change the response they get from adults, teachers and peers.

Make some simple cards with words and phrases from the different ego states of TA:

- critical parent: 'should' 'ought' 'must' 'must not'
- nurturing parent: 'care for' 'look after'
- adult: 'solve' 'co-operative' 'work together'
- free child: 'fun' 'play' 'whoopee' 'no I won't'
- adapted child: 'please' 'may I'

Have some blank paper to add your client's own words.

If your client is in a challenging relationship with family or school, you can offer a new way of understanding what is happening by explaining that using certain words will bring about a particular response. A teenager going home and saying to a surprised parent that they want to solve the problem of who cleans up rather than saying 'you should do it' or 'I won't' to their parent may get an immediately changed response from that parent.

Young children who don't say please or thank you are often criticised or what they want can be withheld. In counselling, you can allow their feelings to be expressed as it may be no more than a convention of language and underlying anger and resentment can be explored. Through understanding how simply changing words and their accompanying gestures or tone of voice may bring resolution of conflict, perhaps a negative 'cycle' of communication can be changed.

An activity like this is used in the spirit of exploration, *never* to criticise or make someone change. The young have lots of times that they need to or must comply in their lives, so they may need encouragement and time to trust that their counsellor is not going to be like that. Some young clients look blank at first when offered choice as this is so unfamiliar to them.

Strengths of integrative approaches

The strength of the integrative counsellor is that they have learnt how to draw together strands of different theories and put them into practice as a coherent 'whole'. An integrative counsellor should have a strong rationale for what is included in their own model of counselling. From this basis, new material can be included when counselling the young client and this may be drawn from any part of this chapter.

COGNITIVE–BEHAVIOURAL

Strengths of CBT approaches

Many aspects of CBT are well suited to young clients. CBT counsellors working with children and young people recognise that there may be distortions in thinking processes and behaviours that are very unhelpful to young clients. CBT counsellors will be able to engage in activities and exercises that help in thinking clearly or modifying behaviour. Goal setting and measuring progress are useful strategies that youngsters often enjoy. If you are a CBT practitioner, it is probable that you will be focusing primarily on the present and future in your counselling, whilst recognising that unhelpful 'negative automatic thinking' is rooted in early experiences.

CBT tends to be goal orientated with an emphasis on change. An extension for those trained in CBT would be to consider the early attachments, or lack of them, that have been made by the young client. It would be inappropriate to ask a child to attempt to analyse how their home life and early attachments are influencing them. As practitioners though, we can gain a lot of useful understanding through conversations with young clients about the family they are growing up in. An absence of feelings about early experiences can also give us lots of information.

An example of this is a 16-year-old young man experiencing severe panic attacks, where nothing in his recent life offers any explanation for the panic. When exploring with him the family he grew up in, the story of his mother's death comes clearly into focus, though it is spoken of without emotion. The client's mother died in a car crash. This client was also in the car as a very young child but remembers nothing of events. His father carried on working full time to support him and various family members helped out whilst he was growing up.

He has never experienced any panic symptoms before or deep upset relating to his mother's death and he tells you the story of this early loss in a distant way, as if he is speaking about the life of someone else. This early childhood trauma is clearly very significant and may well be the reason for the client's current vulnerability and sense of panic.

Whilst we cannot be sure that his witnessing of his mother's death is causing the present panic attacks, it needs to be considered as a factor in understanding this young man's situation. It is not necessary or advisable to dwell on his mother's death in counselling as he remembers so little about it, but holding an awareness of his vulnerability due to the circumstances of the death of his mother may be a vital aspect of the counselling.

Extending CBT training: exploring a young client's early life

1 Drawing a lifeline

This can be done simply on an A4 sheet of paper with one pen or pencil, or it can be done on a large sheet of paper with coloured pens and crayons. How you carry out the exercise will depend on:

- the age and developmental stage of your client
- the context of the counselling
- your own experience with art materials.

Draw a lifeline for your own life as a way to practise before attempting this with a client. On the paper, draw a line that represents your life from birth (or before – it may start at conception) and then begin to write or draw all the events you want to include between then and now; more significant events can be larger to emphasise them. Take as much time as you need. You can use different coloured pens for pleasant and unpleasant memories of events. Be as creative or as simple as you wish. Once the lifeline is drawn, there can be a discussion about what it was like to put this down on paper. Sometimes insights are immediate; in other cases, the drawing may be enough and the relevance of certain memories may not seem significant straightaway.

Once you have completed your own lifeline, you will have more understanding of the kind of impact it may have on young clients.

When using the lifeline method with young clients:

- go at the client's pace – the lifeline may be completed in 10 minutes or take more than one full session of counselling to complete
- express interest in what has been put on the lifeline but don't try and interpret/analyse it
- say what you notice, e.g. 'I notice there is a gap between three and seven years where you didn't put anything on your lifeline'
- don't say: 'You probably don't remember that time in your life because… (you didn't like school/you were jealous of the birth of your sibling/your parents divorced)'; these may be true statements, but children and young people need to find their own meaning
- explore what your client has included in their lifeline
- if you don't understand what has been written or illustrated, ask for clarification, e.g. 'Who is in this picture you have drawn?'
- listen, reflect and be patient – you can keep the lifeline on file and return to it in later sessions
- share puzzles or concerns about the lifeline in supervision – your supervisor can look at it and fresh insights may arise
- don't try to solve all the client's problems through this method, but treat it as part of the ongoing counselling
- remember to focus on positives as well as negatives – it's great to be able to celebrate achievements and joyful moments with young clients
- even if something on a lifeline seems obvious to you, it may be a surprise or shock to your client, so make sure you have enough time to process the activity.

2 Examining or describing a family photo

This is another good way to learn more about the client's family. It may be that what you learn is information about the 'family system' in which the young client lives; as with the lifeline, let the client offer information about the photo, who is in it and who took it. Don't offer your opinion, for instance avoiding statements like 'you look/sad/happy/worried in the photo'; it is better to ask your client what they see and how they were feeling when the photo was taken.

An example of this is Tim, aged 10, who, you have been told, has just witnessed the very difficult marriage break-up of his parents. His father has been having an affair and, you are told by his school link person, there have been aggressive arguments as his father has moved into another building on the farm where they live. During the course of counselling, Tim's father moves away and Tim sees very little of him. Tim brings in a photo showing himself, his dogs who he loves and his older brother who is 18. His mum had taken the photo on a recent day out. Since Tim's dad left, his mum has been very kind and attentive to him, his brother has taken him out more and his mum has been very clear in telling him that it's 'no one's fault' that dad has left: 'these things happen' and 'your dad still loves you'.

When you talk about the photo, Tim is very happy and excited, as he has just got a new puppy and been to his favourite places. Although the impact of Tim's father leaving might be profound in the long term, right now he is enjoying life and is very cheerful.

This kind of situation reminds counsellors that sometimes we are doing preparatory work with children and young people. Making sure that Tim is heard and accepted, even if you are left with concerns that he has not expressed anything about the impact of the marital problems and his father's absence, can mean he will be happy to return to counselling later on if necessary. You can just draw attention to the father's absence, saying that you notice he hasn't mentioned his dad. If he very brightly says, 'oh, dad doesn't live with us now', and if you then ask him how he feels about that and he tells you it's OK because his mum is feeling better now and that makes him happy, then accept this as it is and join with the current feeling of happiness. As counsellors, we don't need to 'water the seeds' of unhappiness or fear in young clients. Conversely, if we sense there is suppression of certain emotions, for example, if, in a particular family, feeling unhappy or crying is not allowed, then education in emotional literacy can be very helpful (there is more on this later in the chapter).

3 Drawing up a family tree or genogram

This can be an essential exercise when there is a complex family system – there may be half siblings and/or step siblings and more than one person that the client thinks of as 'mum' or 'dad' due to multiple changes in home life, so much so that you find it really hard to understand who's who and how they 'fit' together as a family. Writing everyone's name down and working out the family relationships can be made into an interesting activity.

Sometimes I will get clients to test my memory, saying, 'Your dad was married twice before and you have grown-up sisters called Sally and Kim. Kim is now married to Tony and they have got a baby girl called Lisa. Your mum was married once before and Aaron and Michael live with you but have a different dad and his name is Mark. Mark is now married to Eva and they have a daughter ... ohhh, I can't remember her name but she is the same age as you!'

Often, young clients will think it is fun to correct and remind you. The complex families they live in are normal to them and can work very well. At other times, children feel dislocated and don't even know where they are going 'home' to after counselling if their parents have separate homes. There can also be different 'rules' and 'boundaries' provided by two parents who both have new families; this can be very confusing for young clients. They may fall behind with their school work because books they need are in the 'other' house and they can't do their homework. On occasion, one parent wants the child to attend counselling but the other parent objects to it.

All this can be revealed by drawing a family tree or, as in the next exercise, by using small objects to represent family members.

4 Using stones, shells or other small objects to represent 'the family'

Having a good collection of stones, shells or other small objects is very useful for counsellors. As before, try this yourself first, or with another counsellor, to find out how it works in practice. This is an exercise that can be used with adults too and can be particularly good with adolescents who don't want to talk much about their families.

With younger children, it can be introduced as 'making a picture story of the people you live with and other people who are in your family'. Let your client just play with the stones, feeling their texture, looking at the colours, comparing sizes and shapes. Very occasionally, a young client may throw the stones around. There does need to be a safety boundary if this happens. Other objects would be more appropriate in such a case: a selection of small plastic animals can be fun. (See also the use of miniature animals in Chapter 7.)

For example, someone difficult in a child's life might be a fierce tiger and a frightened child could show this by using a mouse to represent themselves. Plenty of variety and enough objects for the young client to choose from would be very helpful.

- Ask your client to choose an object to represent themselves.

- Tell them that they can place the object anywhere in a given space, on a table top or a section of the floor.

- Suggest that they now choose objects to 'be' other people in their lives and put them anywhere in the same area.

- Notice if the objects are close together or far apart: are siblings all lined up in a row? Is the object your client has chosen for themselves big or small in comparison to the others?

- Ask if there is anyone else they would like to put in the 'picture' (it is possible your client will want to put you in).

- Accept the picture they have made and ask what they notice when they look at it.

- Make a few comments about what you notice, e.g. 'I notice you have put your stone very near the one that you put in as your dad, but your mum's stone is much further away from you. The stone you chose for your mum's boyfriend is right in front of your mum's stone. If you were the size of this stone, you might not be able to see your mum very easily as she is right behind her boyfriend in your picture.'

- Never criticise or disbelieve the picture; it's easy to say, 'well, you haven't used many stones' or 'Finished already? Did you really think about this?' These kinds of comments imply that the client has done it wrong. If the client is not very engaged that's OK – it's all voluntary anyway and won't work for every child and young person.
- Don't say 'you need to put in a stone for your brother/gran', etc. If a person is absent from the picture, then that is how your client sees it right now.
- When a young client is very engaged with the exercise, you can ask: 'If I gave you a magic wand and now you can change some stones, where would you move them?'

Keep a note of these exercises as they offer up so much of what you don't immediately see in the counselling room. They give your client a route to telling you about their life without you having to rely on the words they say. Children and young people are usually growing up inside a family that they just accept as the 'norm' – just like we breathe oxygen or a fish lives in water, the young may live in homes where violence, aggression, depression or anxiety are normal everyday occurrences.

It is for this reason that 'anger management' exercises, for example, can be a limited way of helping young clients. It is good for them to learn to manage their own feelings and this can solve their problem in some cases. Often though, youngsters are severely provoked by their home lives, even though families may be doing their best. Patterns of challenging behaviour will keep repeating because a youngster cannot move away from a family life where they experience over-anxiety, rejection, deep criticism or hostility on a daily basis. As Violet Oaklander reminds us:

> The child is provoked by the environment rather than their internal difficulties. What s/he lacks is the ability to cope with an environment that makes her/him angry and fearful. These behaviours that are often considered by adults to be antisocial are often actually a desperate attempt to re-establish a social connection. (1988: 207)

This does not, of course, mean we should blame tired, anxious parents who just see the untidy room and shout or angry parents who see one of their children as 'the cause of all their problems'. Our anger will not help the situation. Even though we may not be able to enter into any kind of relationship with the young client's family, as counsellors of the young we need to understand as much as we can about their life outside of the counselling room.

The exercises above will help us to gain the 'child's eye view' of their life. Once we have an understanding of the challenges our clients face on a daily basis, there is the opportunity to offer strategies towards improving their family relationships. Most important though is to be alongside them in their daily trials. Kindness, connection and approval help to build a youngster's resilience and a sense that they are, in many cases, not at fault when they act up in the difficult family circumstances they were born into. Often, it is really difficult for a child to 'get it right' in families where there is substance misuse, severe financial problems or a lack of time to give attention. Overprotection, anxiety and stress in the family can also lead to behaviour in the young that is troubling. Trying to stop these behaviours may be necessary for social inclusion, but, for counselling, the depth of relationship can bring about a change in the way young clients feel about themselves, leading to changes in behaviour that will last.

Simply smiling at a young client, noticing what they are doing well, taking the time to get to know them is likely to make a difference in how they behave both with you and outside of counselling; be honest, too, if you think they are causing themselves problems through challenging behaviours, always focusing on the behaviour as separate from who they are. It's so common to see a child or young person as 'angry' or 'withdrawn'. Labels like 'she never listens' or 'he is always naughty' don't give much room for the change process. Counsellors have the time and opportunity to get to know the young client and suddenly the reason for their behaviour becomes clear.

Fortunately, this connection and understanding can be enough to reduce challenging behaviour in many young clients; once they are feeling a bit better about themselves, they can manage to be quieter in class or less furious with a younger sibling, or when they are told to be quiet and it was actually someone else talking, they can move on without having to scream and cry and get into more trouble. I expect most of us can remember being misjudged or misunderstood as children. If there is no one to support us on these occasions and there are punishments that hurt, who wouldn't feel angry or sad? Young children learn through imitation. Learning about your client's home life and past experiences is crucial to understanding their current situation and helps to piece together reasons why certain unhelpful behaviours have formed.

Aspects of CBT that are particularly helpful with young clients

- Scaling – regularly checking how a young client is feeling on a scale of 1 to 10, 1 being really not good and 10 being excellent, is a very good intervention and can be used with youngsters of any age. An unusual result of using this technique with younger children is that they will often go outside the scale. Hearing that a young child feels 'minus a million' is not uncommon, even if the request has been to place themselves on a scale between 1 and 10.

- 'That's just the way your brain works and it's not your fault' can be a very useful intervention. This idea comes from 'compassion-focused therapy', a branch of CBT (Gilbert 2010) that helps us understand how our bodies respond to feeling threatened and will cause us to behave in certain ways that are not our fault. This 'no-blame' approach can be particularly helpful with teenagers who are often blamed and criticised quite heavily for behaviours that are connected with their developmental stage. Recent research has shown that teenagers benefit greatly from being allowed to sleep in the mornings because of aspects of their brain function. Based on research, some schools in the USA and one in England are now starting classes at 10.00 am to enable teenagers to be more focused and less sleepy in class. Better exam results have been the outcome of this change (see www.sleepfoundation.org).

PSYCHODYNAMIC

Strengths of the psychodynamic approach

A focus on early attachment and loss is an aspect of psychodynamic training that is central for counselling young clients. As was explained in Chapter 1, culturally our view of children has been altered through the contribution of Bowlby, recognising the child's need for a secure base and the likely outcomes if there is not enough secure attachment at a very young age. Physiologically, a baby develops differently if there is a lack of attachment. There has been evidence to show that brain development changes if there is a lack of affection and continuity in infancy, so attachment to the primary caregiver is now accepted as necessary for healthy development rather than being 'nice to have'.

For those trained to connect with unconscious processes and work through transference, the speed and lightness often present in counselling children and young people can present a challenge. You may be fortunate to be placed in a clinic or in private practice where there is the opportunity to unfold the counselling over a long period of time. Many contexts, however, will want lots of clients to have the chance to see you and long-term work may only be possible with a minority of clients or not at all.

Young clients, too, sometimes want to just pop in or are sent by adults and don't really engage in any depth. Further, traumatised children may need to focus on managing their present-day circumstances as any remembering of the past is likely to be too painful and difficult for them.

An example of this is counselling a child or young person who has been involved in a tragic event. These events occur everywhere. Counsellors have experienced cases where children and young people have:

- witnessed the suicide or murder of siblings
- cared for a dying friend
- tried to save a drowning friend who died
- witnessed a friend fall under a train whilst playing together on a railway line.

These cases are often unforgettable and shocking for all involved. In some cases, the young client speaks very little, if at all, about the tragedy in counselling.

The issue for the counsellor is that understanding the consequences of these circumstances does not change the fact that young clients may not be ready, willing or able to discuss their past.

Extending psychodynamic training

Making here-and-now relationships after tragic events

- In the first session, allow the client to talk about the tragic event if they wish to.
- If they don't mention the tragedy, let them know that you know about what happened.
- Explain that people are concerned that they may be feeling upset or frightened, having dreams or nightmares.
- Sometimes clients will begin to talk about how they are feeling; in many cases, though, their concerns are about schoolwork, how upset their mum has been or just wanting to move on.
- Allow the client to use the session to speak about what is bothering them in the here and now.
- Don't keep referring back to the incident if the client doesn't want to talk further about it.
- Let a reparative and welcoming relationship develop between you in the present.
- Play and laugh together if this is what the client wants.
- Be encouraging and let the client know you notice that they are managing well.
- Say that one day you think they may want to talk further about the tragic event, but whether they do so or not is entirely their choice.
- Let them know that what happened was in NO way their fault and then don't refer to what happened again unless they do.

Psychodynamic counsellors can usefully extend into emotional literacy education with young clients.

Activity: Naming the feeling

Adults and children alike often don't know what it is they are feeling. In my practice with adults, I will sometimes say: 'Feelings are often expressed in short words: happy, sad, cross, fed up, joy, glee, etc., in response to a long, convoluted description as to what is "going on" for them.' With groups of children and young people, even with those of a similar age, there can be widely differing views as to what a feeling is. In school groups, I have heard some youngsters aged 8–10 offer up a good understanding of subtle feelings like envy, when others of the same age are looking bemused.

It's a good idea to at least check that your client has the language available to them to express how they feel.

Naming feelings with children aged 11 and under:

- Show the young client a range of pictures of children whose facial expressions show how they are feeling.
- Rather than telling the child 'this is a happy face', ask them what they see.
- When they have identified a feeling (it may be a different one to the answer you expected), ask if they have ever felt like this and whether they can tell you about it.
- Try giving your own examples, e.g. 'I often feel happy in the sunshine on the beach by the sea' or 'I felt sad when my grandma died'. This gives permission for feelings to be spoken.

Sometimes there is one feeling that is more risky for children, and often this is anger. Helping young children to understand that it is possible to feel anger without punching or exploding can be helpful.

- It can be OK to feel anger, but it's more tricky for children as they are often not allowed to 'walk away' from a situation. They have to stay in class or in the room with an aggressive sibling, for example. How do they cope?
- Conversations about feelings with young children can give them 'tools' to recognise and accept that feelings are allowed.

Naming feelings with young people aged 11–15:

- Encourage this age group to use whatever language they need to in order to express themselves, as long as it's not offensive to you.
- Be aware that if a youngster says they feel 'shit', this could mean so many different things.
- Ask them what kind of 'shit' they feel. Often, the surprise they experience at you accepting their language allows them to expand and explain, being the 'expert' on their own feelings.
- Note that the same applies to them telling you they feel 'cool', 'rubbish', 'crap' or 'wicked' or any other colloquial expression that is common in their peer group.
- Appreciate that this is an exercise in mutual understanding – you enter into the client's world, accepting that this is their language, without judging, then you ask them to expand on and widen their understanding of what it means to them to be feeling like that.
- Prepare to hear something that you personally find unacceptable. For me, it's OK whatever a young person's swearing is like, as long as it's not aimed at me. Swearing at me, calling me names is not acceptable. This needs to be made clear, as once you take the lid off the modified language youngsters use with adults in authority, lots can come out.
- Say: 'So what is feeling "crap" like for you?' Enter into the discovery of feelings and give clients the chance to become more emotionally literate.

Naming feelings with 15–18-year-olds:

The exercise above for 11–15s may help this age group as well – as the young person makes the transition to the adult world, they need to understand how to express emotions in a healthy way.

- Explain that recognising and managing feelings is a skill, just like other skills – if they didn't know how to use their mobile phones well, they wouldn't be able to communicate with their friends. They had to learn how to use technology and now there is an opportunity to learn to be skilful with feelings.
- Open up discussion about personal relationships, this age group can get completely tongue-tied when wanting to speak with someone they feel attracted to.
- If young clients are comfortable then go deeper with questions such as: What did you actually feel? Shame, inadequacy, fear or shyness? What happens in your body when you feel shy – for example, blushing, feeling 'rooted to the spot' or covering it all up with shows of over-loud boisterous behaviour?
- Consider that this discussion about feelings in personal relationships may be useful with some under-15s too.

Discussions like this mean that the counsellor needs to be comfortable in expressing feelings and talking through potentially embarrassing subjects. It often involves humour and a light yet intimate counselling relationship.

Never push at these topics, but if they can be opened up they will give permission for the inner world of the teenager to be included in the counselling. Often, 'pushing' can be the way of a counsellor coping with the feeling of 'dissatisfaction when they experience the young person's resistance' (Reid and Westergaard 2011: 120). The pushing feels helpful to the counsellor but will probably mean that the young person closes down and feels defensive.

Being involved and self-disclosure

With children and young people, there are ways in which we are more involved than when with adults. We maintain our professional role, the same as with any client, and rely on our training and position as counsellor to inform the choice of interventions made. We are, however, responsible for the well-being of young clients in a way that we are not with adults. Adults at risk require deep consideration, and often counsellors will discuss with their supervisor if any action needs to be taken to make sure they are safe. In most cases, their autonomy is primary unless they are at immediate risk of death or serious injury. With children and young people, it is vital to maintain confidentiality where it is safe to do so. There are, however, some cases where the need to safeguard a child has to take precedence over the need for confidentiality. This will be examined in depth in the following chapter.

Self-disclosure can be very helpful in forming the therapeutic alliance; this does not mean 'baring your soul' to your client, rather letting them know that you were young once and remember what it was like. In this context, it is a form of empathy to say:

- I felt angry at school.
- My sister got more attention sometimes, because she was younger and not well.
- I had to give away my dog and felt sad for ages.
- I wasn't good at PE.

When you have had vastly different life experiences to your client, you can say 'I don't know anything about that. What is it like to:

- be the fifth child in a family?
- have two parents living in different countries?
- feel excluded from your friends on internet sites?
- live with foster families?
- win a prize at school, but have no one you know turn up to the ceremony when you receive it?'

Whatever your young client's life is like, they may be glad on occasion to know that yours was not plain sailing, that you got into trouble at school or had a girlfriend/boyfriend who 'dumped' you. The fact that you are now a counsellor and got past the child/adolescent difficulties and got a job may be very welcome news. In adolescence particularly, difficulties can seem entirely overwhelming and 'global', there being no sense that they will pass. A measured self-disclosure – one that you know will not impact too heavily if the client questions you about it – can be highly facilitative to the counselling relationship.

PERSON-CENTRED AND HUMANISTIC

Strengths of person-centred and humanistic approaches

Counsellors who are person-centred and humanistic will value the relationship and be comfortable with allowing the young client's agenda to be expressed. Non-directive play therapy is a very good example of how to translate the person-centred approach into work with children. In *Play Therapy* (1947/1989), Virginia Axline outlined the principles of non-directive play therapy – these principles still stand today as an excellent foundation for counselling children:

1. The therapist develops a warm, friendly relationship with the child.
2. The therapist accepts the child exactly as they are.
3. The therapist establishes a feeling of permissiveness in the relationship.
4. The therapist is alert to recognising the feelings that a child is expressing and reflects those back to them to gain insight.

5. The therapist maintains a deep respect for the child's ability to solve their own problems.
6. The therapist does not attempt to direct the child's conversation or actions in any manner.
7. The therapist does not attempt to hurry the therapy along.
8. The therapist establishes only those limitations that are necessary to anchor the therapy in the world of reality.

Axline's extended case study of Dibs (1964) offers clear insight into this method of action. At the beginning of her first session of play therapy with Dibs, Axline writes:

> We had an hour to spend in this room. There was no urgency to get anything done. To play or not to play. To talk or to be silent, in here it would make no difference. (1964: 22)

Oaklander gives many examples of creative ways to be with children in a Gestalt, humanistic framework. She writes:

> I want them [children] to know that they have choices about how they will live in their world, how they will react to it, how they will manipulate it. I cannot presumptuously make this choice for them. I can only do my part to give them the strength to make those choices they want to make and know when choices are impossible to make. (1988: 61)

Extending person-centred and humanistic training

The extension for person-centred counsellors is in accepting that time limitations or the context of counselling children and young people may best be served by more active interventions whilst holding the relationship and being client led.

The proactive approach

Person-centred and humanistic counsellors have an excellent foundation through building relationship for communicating with children and young people. Sometimes the approach is not active enough alone to take into account the way young people are. In a sense, it is person-centred to be more active with young clients as that is a response to how this client group tends to be.

Geldard and Geldard (2010) recommend the proactive approach primarily for adolescents, in order to respond to their developmental stage and need for autonomy and individuation.

Activity for being proactive with young people

Practise allowing a young person to be 'in control' of the conversation and then taking control yourself, and also influence the conversation by introducing a new direction and strategies – this needs to happen in a fluid manner that fits the young style of communication. Young clients often don't like to be told what to do, rather they like choice and a sense of freedom, so responding to different types of open questions may be of value:

- What is happening inside you right now?

- Earlier you talked about your step-father. I am wondering how your brothers and sisters relate to him?

- What would you like to do now? Do you want to change the subject or talk more about this?

- What do you think your life would be like if you didn't feel so resentful?

Geldard and Geldard emphasise that the over-use of questions can result in 'an interrogation not counselling' (2010: 130); conversely, not asking questions and simply responding is often not the best approach and can lead to young clients feeling confused about the counselling process.

Exercises and 'packs'

Recognising that other health professionals, such as school nurses and mentors, have 'stress' and 'anger' packs containing exercises that young clients can work through, it is a good idea for counsellors to know how and when some aspects of these tools may be useful in counselling. Children and young people are very familiar with this way of learning. Of course, it can be completed in an 'on the surface' way without expressing what is going on at a deeper level or being in relationship with the helper.

In counselling, however, if exercises in packs can be brought alive, and be a 'jumping off point' for a deeper discussion of feelings and thoughts, then they can be helpful.

An example of this is the 'blob people' and the 'blob tree' (www.blobtree.com). These are pictures of 'blobby' looking people showing a wide variety of characteristics, ranging from joy to misery, isolation to connection, anger to kindness.

- Give your client a sheet of 'blobs' and ask what they notice.

- Give your client an opportunity to identify themselves or others they know with any of the characters. There may be immediate engagement or a reticence to engage; if it doesn't make sense to your client then they can just leave it. It is simply a route to explaining feelings or situations that your client may not have easy access to the words for.

- If there is an identification – 'that's just like me' or 'that one is how I was before X happened' or 'that's how it is between me and my friends' – explain that this identification can change, maybe in five minutes or far into the future; this is just for now.

- Talk together about what your client sees in the blob picture; don't assume that what they see will be the same as your interpretation of an image.

- Gradually put the picture aside and allow the client to talk further about what has arisen for them.

- Occasionally, refer back to the 'blob' they chose, if appropriate.

- Don't go on to other techniques or pack exercises in the same session, as there can be too much of this in counselling.

- Find humour and fun in the activities, and smile together about the array of blobs and how we all know people like this.

Unintended consequences

Client-centred counsellors who are excellent at joining with their young client's world view may miss the recognition that what is actually happening in the client's life is too risky for them to manage alone. This is where appropriate supervision with a supervisor who is experienced in counselling children and young people becomes such a vital part of the process.

We can become so absorbed in wanting to support our client in what is important to them that a wider view becomes obscured.

Examples of this include the following:

- A young carer, aged 15, who is looking after a parent and younger siblings, doesn't want any outside involvement or support because he fears the family will be broken up and his younger siblings taken into care.

- A 10-year-old, who is experiencing physical punishment on a daily basis, has seen social work interventions in the past and not much has changed at home so the best thing is not to make it worse by telling anyone now.

- A 14-year-old, who feels ready for relationships with older men and is meeting more than one man over 25 years of age, doesn't talk to you about sex but is self-harming by cutting herself.

Reading these, it seems unlikely that anyone would not view these youngsters as being in need of more support than a counsellor can offer in one hour a week. However, when the counsellor forms a deep and trusting relationship with their client, there is the possibility of missing the fact that the client, or others around them, are more at risk than they realise.

Unintended consequences is a very good way to think about this situation as it takes a no-blame approach. In the final example above, we can imagine how a 14-year-old could feel that she was completely in control of her relationships with older men. It is also the case that counsellors must not rush to break confidentiality with young people who have confided in them about their relationships. However, just because a young person feels they are safe it doesn't mean that they are not at risk.

Privacy is necessary for counselling and it is so important that we respect the confidential relationship whilst holding awareness that we may have to go against our client's express wishes in some circumstances because there are likely consequences of their behaviour that they just don't understand. This is NOT the same as automatically reporting confidential material in the case of historical or minor risks. In Chapter 5, we will consider confidentiality in more detail. Disclosure against the client's express wishes is to be recognised as a major step.

The focus here is on recognising that holding the client's world view in a completely person-centred manner may impair the wider world view of risk and likely consequences.

SYSTEMIC

Strengths of systemic counsellors

Our clients often live in complex family systems, with the great majority living inside systems that are not of their own choosing. Systemic counsellors will have an excellent grasp of how the unseen family system the young client lives within is profoundly influencing the way they are developing and acting. Systemic counsellors recognise that what may seem to be dysfunctional or disruptive behaviour in school, may actually be functional to managing a particular home life. There are many cases in which it becomes clear to the counsellor that a child or young person is being 'scapegoated', i.e. they are seen as the reason that there are problems in the family.

It is helpful to that family to have someone to blame and it gives them the opportunity not to consider how they might change themselves, as the problems are seen to reside only in the scapegoat. The difficulties that can arise for a child trapped in the position of the 'bad' or 'wrong' child cannot be overstated. A child can be seen to be born at the wrong time, be the wrong sex or have the wrong looks. Becoming an object of hatred or ridicule is not overstating some cases of this. Parents with these views and opinions about their offspring are very difficult to reach and as counsellors we may never even meet them. We can, however, help to modify the young client's 'internalised' view of themselves.

Extending systemic training

Activity: Use of metaphor and analogy from children's stories

- Sometimes it becomes clear that a parent does not seem to 'see' their child clearly and has very fixed views about them.
- A useful way to explain this is by saying that all of us can have a 'wrong' pair of spectacles on, like in *The Wizard of Oz*, where everyone has to wear green spectacles to maintain the illusion that 'Oz' is a wonderful wizard, when really he's a funny little man with no power.

- Cinderella was a kind person, but her step-mother was jealous and treated her badly – we don't agree with that step-mother's view, do we?

Find the right story to illustrate your particular client's predicament – children's stories are full of examples like this.

Show that you have a different, less biased opinion about the client:

- Give your young client specific examples of behaviour you have witnessed that is not like the idea other adults have about them, e.g. 'I have noticed you turn up on time to counselling so you are not always unreliable.'

- It may be that the client knows there are echoes, resonances and reminders of other family members placed on them; you can then say: 'Just because you look like your dad, it doesn't mean you are exactly like him. Your mum calls your dad "a nightmare" and says you are turning out like him – perhaps she's angry and upset after the divorce? We can all make assumptions or perceive things wrongly sometimes. You are not exactly the same as your dad and both your dad and mum will have some good qualities.'

It is vital to take a 'no-blame' approach to this type of projecting or externalising of the negative. If we then 'blame' the mother, we are just continuing the cycle, the 'blaming culture'. It can be very painful to witness a youngster trying in vain to prove that they are better than their family's negative view of them. As counsellors, we can offer another view, but changing the parent's mind is not in our remit. We would need to consider intervening if the home life was abusive or neglectful, but it may just be sad or confusing. Your client may now be acting in ways that have long been expected of them, complicating the situation. If someone consistently yells at a child or discriminates against them, eventually the child will probably get angry and be unpleasant in return, fuelling the flames of family problems, making the situation a 'self-fulfilling prophecy'.

The counsellor's ability to keep calm and not get pulled into taking sides or rescuing is so important in these types of situations. Sometimes there is a positive 'projection' – the 'golden' child who can do no wrong. This can also cause problems and is part of mistaken perception.

Those trained systemically will recognise that they need to consider the young client in front of them as an individual, a person with their own thoughts, feelings and choices to be made. The systemic perspective is very useful. It would, however, be a mistake to believe it meant making assumptions about who a child or young person is because of the family they grew up in.

NARRATIVE

Strengths of narrative approaches

The narrative approach offers the useful concept that who we are is less 'fixed' than in some other approaches and it views 'problems' as separate from people. Narrative conversations are collaborative and guided by both client and counsellor.

Morgan (undated), as introduced in Chapter 2, gives a clear example of how narrative therapy can change the way events are understood, explaining that we may have a 'thin description' of something that has happened.

Sean, a young man who has been caught stealing, is deemed 'attention seeking' by his family; a story weaved to support this idea of who Sean is leads to the 'thin conclusion' that Sean is 'an attention seeker'. The problem with Sean then gets bigger and bigger and can affect future events. Sean's competencies are then hidden by this definition of who he is. Narrative therapists 'seek out alternative stories' through conversation about how clients would like to live their lives and by discovering, such as in Sean's case, that he is not only attention seeking, but can also give attention, for example. With new stories, Sean can begin to live and understand himself and others in a different way.

Extending narrative training

It may be most useful for narrative counsellors to extend by taking into account that some children and young people are not able to tell their own story very well, if at all, and may not have the ability to participate in verbal re-authoring. This ability is not connected with age as even very young children can create a new story of themselves. Some children and young people, however, cannot or will not talk in this way and an alternative approach is necessary.

No talk therapy

Those who cannot respond to conversation-based therapy can be engaged in various kinds of play and community activities (see Chapter 7 on play). Straus (1999) engages in activities that range from sitting on the floor playing games to helping an adolescent get a job. Whilst this may be outside some counsellors' range, it is useful to consider that the lack of conversation does not have to be the end of counselling.

CHAPTER SUMMARY

This chapter has explored the way in which different theoretical orientations may approach counselling children and young people. It is essential to keep our young clients at the centre of our choices whatever modality we use. The counselling offered needs to be relevant for the challenging circumstances of our clients' lives. The young have resilience and internal resources, but are also vulnerable to being damaged by their environment and circumstances. Through listening to and being with young clients, both within and when extending our theoretical orientation, we will be able to find the flexibility to go beyond what is familiar. Activities such as those in this chapter give us routes to connect deeply in a young-client-centred approach.

REFERENCES

Axline, V. (1947/1989) *Play Therapy*. New York: Ballantine.
Axline, V. (1964) *Dibs in Search of Self*. Harmondsworth: Penguin.
Geldard, K. and Geldard, D. (2010) *Counselling Adolescents*. London: Sage.
Gilbert, P. (2010) *Compassion Focused Therapy*. London: Routledge.
Miller, W.R. and Rollnick, S. (2002) *Motivational Interviewing: Preparing People for Change*, 2nd edn. New York: Guilford Press.
Morgan, A. (undated) An Introduction to Narrative Therapy: The Story of Sean. Available at: www.dulwichcentre.com.au/what-is-narrative-therapy.html
Oaklander, V. (1988) *Windows to Our Children: A Gestalt Therapy Approach to Children and Adolescents*. Moab, UT: Real People Press.
Reid, H.L. and Westergaard, J. (2011) *Effective Counselling with Young People*. Exeter: Learning Matters.
Straus, M. (1999) *No Talk Therapy*. New York: W.W. Norton.

5

SKILLS IN MANAGING PROFESSIONAL ISSUES: CONFIDENTIALITY AND DISCLOSURE, AGREEMENTS AND CONTRACTS

INTRODUCTION

This chapter highlights professional issues that arise when counselling children and young people. Counselling is a private matter and confidentiality needs to be maintained. In exceptional cases though, disclosures may need to be made when a young client does not want this.

Becoming a skilled practitioner when clients are 'minors' in legal terms, involves familiarity with relevant laws that influence whether confidentiality can be maintained or not. Counsellors are often managers of the boundary between confidentiality and disclosure with a child or young person.

Parents/carers, teachers and other professionals may share information about a child or young person's life in order to keep them safe. Your young client, however, has disclosed to you in confidence and has a right to expect privacy. This potential conflict of interest can arise on a daily basis when counselling children and young people. Counsellors need to understand what influences the confidential service that can be offered.

In this chapter, we will explore:

- confidentiality and disclosure
- explaining to parents/carers about confidentiality in counselling
- the legal framework
- Gillick competence
- when consent is needed
- agreements and contracts.

> ### MINDFUL MOMENT: RESPONDING TO PROFESSIONAL ISSUES
>
> Take a moment to breathe quietly and notice how the issues listed above affect you.
>
> Do you enjoy thinking about the legal framework, confidentiality and disclosure or does it bring anxieties and fears to mind? Note your responses and consider how to find the best way in yourself to manage these issues well. Recognise that you do not need to be alone with any decisions you make about disclosure or conflicts of interest.
>
> Breathe in and out evenly and recognise your best way to manage professional issues. Know that you can return to this quiet moment if tensions build up when resolving challenging professional issues.

CONFIDENTIALITY AND DISCLOSURE

The confidential nature of counselling with children and young people marks the profession as separate from others in the helping professions (Bond and Mitchels 2008). We are in a similar position to doctors in that we need to hold what our young clients tell us as private and confidential unless there are exceptional reasons – usually the risk of significant harm – that require us to disclose. Where the risk of significant harm exists, sharing information is in the best interests of our clients, as keeping them safe must be the priority. In practice, risk of significant harm can be much more difficult to discern than we might imagine, particularly if our client is no longer at risk but other children are at risk in a disclosed situation. We may need to break our client's confidentiality to keep others safe.

Other professionals, social workers, health visitors and teachers often prioritise sharing information in order to keep a child or young person safe. As counsellors, we need to explain our approach to confidentiality when we are questioned or given information about young clients: 'There is a growing body of research evidence which demonstrates the vital importance to children and young people of confidentiality, as a critical factor influencing their decision to disclose sensitive personal information' (Daniels and Jenkins 2010: 55).

For some readers, there will be puzzlement at the reasons that counsellors won't keep confidentiality with children and young people. Some counsellors initially hold the view that there is really no difference from adults when considering the confidential counselling relationship. In reality, the situation is very different when the client is a child or young person. Keeping confidentiality with young clients is a complex matter.

Many people believe that children and young people are the responsibility of their parents/carers until they reach the age of 18. For those who hold this belief, it follows that, for this responsibility to be carried out fully, parents/carers need to be aware of everything their children are doing/thinking/feeling.

Counsellors will meet the situation where parents don't want their children to have confidential counselling because of:

- the possibility of being accused of abuse or neglect
- criminal activity in the home, such as illegal drug use
- feeling guilty, ashamed or upset about problems in the family
- holding a strong belief that family matters remain private
- a mistrust or misunderstanding of what counselling is.

Conversely, some parents want to know what their children say in counselling in order to protect or help them. Some parents want so much involvement that they give lots of information to the counsellor. If parents/carers are distressed, they may need to get support from friends, family or their GP or have their own counselling. Counsellors need to maintain focus on their young client.

As counsellors of the young, we need to keep our client's position central in our thinking, feeling and actions. This means holding a child and young person centred approach whilst being non-judgemental towards parents/carers. We know that, unfortunately, some parents/carers do not act in their child's best interests. There is a need to be discerning and ready to act if abuse or neglect is revealed. Be sure you know the procedure for skilful disclosure within the context you are counselling.

Parents/carers will sometimes expect you to join them in conversation about their child. Depending on the circumstances and age of your client, choose carefully how you respond.

It is crucial that you do not allow yourself to be rushed or persuaded by anyone to disclose information about your client unthinkingly.

You need to be aware of how strange and new it is for parents/carers to be excluded from knowing about their child. Confidentiality with us as counsellors may mean separation and loss from an intimate space between parent and child, as well as fears about how they will be represented by their offspring in counselling.

If you are or have been a parent/carer yourself, imagine what it would be like to know your child was distressed and that someone else knew about it and you did not. Some parents/carers are very happy or even grateful that their child has someone else to talk to. Others want to respect confidentiality, but may want to give information or ask questions too.

Parents/carers and other adults may invite you to 'collude' in the sense of saying, 'I know it's all confidential, but [the client] doesn't need to know that we are having a little chat; it's "off the record"'. This type of approach is very tempting for the counsellor who wants a good relationship with the adults in their young client's life. Resisting the invitation to chat about your young client whilst maintaining excellent, co-operative relationships with adults in their life 'informally', is a tremendously important skill and one that needs to be cultivated.

Situations often arise quite suddenly where challenges are made to the confidential relationship. Counsellors may be approached in the following way.

CASE EXAMPLE: MEETING A CLIENT'S MOTHER UNEXPECTEDLY

Carl's mother asks you: 'How is Carl getting on in counselling? He's a nightmare at home', and then says: 'Did you know that Carl's sister is very ill and is undergoing more tests? Does he talk about that in counselling?'

This type of questioning and information giving can be difficult to respond to. In this case, Carl's mum who wants to talk to you about her son who is 14, most probably thinks she is being helpful and interested.

There are occasions as counsellors when we do need to know something our client has not told us. More often than not though, this type of intervention is not helpful for counsellors. Once you have been told something, you cannot pretend you do not know it as this may affect your ability to be present and congruent with your client.

Being polite and letting parents/carers know that it is best for us to hear about a client's life from the client requires diplomacy and skill. In the case of the first question, 'How is Carl getting on in counselling?', asked by Carl's mum, one response is: 'If you want to know how Carl is getting on in counselling, then it's best to ask him.' This response may put Carl under pressure if Carl's mum then goes to Carl and says: 'Your counsellor wants you to talk to me about how you are getting on in counselling.' Carl may then come to counselling and say: 'Why did you expect me to tell my mum what we are talking about?'

It is therefore better to address the issue of confidentiality with Carl's mum: 'I need to keep what is said in counselling confidential as Carl is my client. If there is any possibility of significant harm to him then I will talk the matter through with Carl and then let you know. Counselling often works best if the confidential relationship is allowed to develop. It's best if I don't hear about his life from you or tell you how he is getting on in counselling.' You may want to add information about supervision and how you review your casework with your supervisor.

Later, when you see Carl again, let him know that you have re-affirmed the boundaries of confidentiality with his mother. By only giving factual information to his mum about the framework of counselling and maintaining a professional manner, you have protected the confidential relationship. Emphasise to Carl that you did not and will not disclose anything of what has been said in counselling unless he or others he has spoken of are in danger of significant harm. Even if a disclosure becomes necessary, it would be good practice to discuss it with Carl first.

The need to reiterate the nature of the confidential relationship is a major aspect of being a child and young person's counsellor.

EXPLAINING TO PARENTS/CARERS ABOUT CONFIDENTIALITY IN COUNSELLING

Children NOT competent to consent to counselling

There needs to be an agreement or 'consent form' for the parent/guardian if a young client is not able or allowed to consent to counselling themselves. Often, a distinction about who consents is made in terms of whether the child is in primary or secondary education. If the child is at primary school, up to age 11, consent from a person with parental responsibility is often automatically sought and children accept this as the 'norm' in their life that an adult decides for them in these types of situations. A counsellor based in primary education will often be told that there is a potential client, but that they can't yet be seen as a consent form has not been completed.

Children in year 6, the final year in primary education where children are 10 and 11 years old, can make very good use of counselling. Children of this age are unlikely to be considered competent to consent in law, according to the Children's Legal Centre (1997). Their development will vary but some children of this age would be competent to consent to counselling. In most cases, however, the practicalities mean that parental consent will need to be obtained. This does not mean that parents have an automatic right to know what the child is discussing in counselling. Often, parents/carers are supportive and welcome the opportunity for their child to be counselled.

The consent form can be brief, just asking the parent/carer to give their agreement for counselling to take place, with a sentence about confidentiality and its limits. It can be a good idea to simply give all parents/carers a leaflet about all the services available to children and young people in the community centre and include counselling in the list of services. It should be made clear that this information alone does not constitute informed consent.

Young people competent to consent to counselling

There can be concerns expressed by parents/carers about needing to know what is going on with their child, even when the child is competent to consent to confidential counselling. This impulse to be included needs to be understood by the counsellor and managed in a way that encourages confidence in the counselling process.

The schools counselling toolkit (BACP/WAG undated) offers an example of an information sheet that can be given to parents/carers:

Is it confidential?

A key feature of our service is that information discussed in the counselling session is treated confidentially. Counselling is a time when it's OK to talk about concerns without fear of them being discussed elsewhere. This includes not discussing the work with parents, unless the child or young person requests or gives consent for this. This can be hard for parents to accept at times, but ensuring the confidentiality of the work is crucial for establishing trust so that the children and young people feel confident to speak openly and freely about what is concerning them.

However, if a pupil appears to be at risk of significant harm it may be appropriate to seek help from other agencies to keep them safe. The counsellor would aim to discuss this first with the pupil concerned. All counsellors receive supervision of their work with young people, to ensure the quality of their practice and this is confidential.

What if I don't want my child to receive counselling?

If a child or young person requests counselling and is able to understand what is involved in the process, then they have the right to access counselling. Parents/carers may not deny them this right. We would, however, prefer that we have your support for the work, and we are always happy to talk with you about any concerns that you may have about the idea of counselling.

This excerpt gives us a sense of how important it is to explain and hold the boundaries of counselling with children and young people, whatever the context of that counselling.

Counsellors know there are very good reasons for confidentiality and we need to be clear about what the purposes are. There is also a need to understand that from the parent/carer's point of view, keeping confidentiality can seem strange and unnecessary. When a young person receives confidential counselling, it may be the first time that anything has been kept from their parents/carers. Parents/carers can respond in a wide variety of ways, from being grateful that their child has someone whom they feel able to confide in, to feeling angry and shut out. It is very important for counsellors with young clients to learn how to conduct contact with parents/carers skilfully and non-judgementally. It is easy for counsellors to ascribe challenging behaviour in their clients to dysfunctions in others who care for them. We know, of course, that the young client's home life deeply influences their well-being or lack of it. A calm, professional approach to all those involved in the life of the young client is essential, whether this is re-affirming the confidential nature of counselling or making arrangements for attendance at future sessions. These skills are an integral part of counselling children and young people.

Skills in communication with parents/carers

Sometimes the first person you speak to about a young client is an adult who wants them to have counselling. Be prepared to discuss the counselling whilst not becoming too involved in their view of the young client. It's best to keep an open mind about your new young client when you meet them for the first time.

With the 'referring' adult, communications include:

Progress not process

If a parent/carer or teacher asks how a child is progressing, you can offer statements like: 'Andy is engaged and co-operative' or 'Rima wants to continue with counselling;

I think she needs to come for another five sessions'. Parents/carers may be paying for the counselling or investing time and effort in getting their child to sessions. They need to know basic factual information. The main way they will know about how effective the counselling is will be by noticing changes in their child.

Establishing the boundaries

The counselling is not for the parent/carer. Sometimes there is confusion about this when the adult who is organising the counselling wants to be in the sessions and does need support because the child's issues are profoundly affecting them. Be clear who the counselling is for. Referral to a family therapist may be appropriate if the whole family wants to be involved in the counselling process. Referral to another counsellor for the parent/carer may also be helpful.

Parents/carers in the counselling room

If your client is a younger child, someone coming into the counselling room with them is appropriate at first. The boundary of that person leaving the room needs to be established from the first session. There needs to be flexibility according to the needs of your client, rather than the needs of the parent/carer, though sometimes it is difficult to discern at first whose need it is for the adult to be there.

Arriving and leaving

The importance of adhering to start and collection times must be explained if a child or young person is counselled in private practice. Having a child in a waiting room when you need to start another session is not acceptable. An excellent example of this can be seen in the case of 'Oliver' in the US TV series *In Treatment* (HBO 2012). It is unpleasant for all if the adult who is bringing the child to counselling is consistently late in collecting them. If this does happen, find a way to talk to the person at another time about the need to be on time when arriving and leaving.

Mutual respect

Always maintain a respectful approach towards a parent/carer, even when you have just heard from your young client about injustices or upsetting events in their home life. Parents/carers are doing their best and they are bringing their child to counselling. A counsellor can also expect respect from the parent/carer and needs to understand their stress whilst not allowing any venting of anger or other unacceptable behaviour by the parent/carer in the counselling room.

Counsellors' independence

Counsellors with children and young people need to explain why they are not going to chat or become too friendly with parents/carers. It may be obvious to you and a complete mystery to your client's parents/carers or teachers why you maintain a professional approach.

Talking to adults when the young client is present

Do not be drawn into conversation with parents/carers or teachers about your client. If you need to pass on factual information, times of sessions, etc., do so politely and professionally. Questions you may be asked include: 'How is s/he getting on?' This can then be usefully discussed with your client: 'Your mum wants to know how you are getting on in counselling; shall we invite her in for 10 minutes next time to discuss progress?' or 'I might speak on the phone to your dad to discuss progress; I won't be talking to him about your feelings or any subjects we have discussed'. Give examples to your client of what you might say. You may sometimes need to listen to the views of parents/carers. It's important never to do this with the child present 'as if' they were not there. Edges of confidentiality are very easily compromised in these situations.

REFLECTIVE ACTIVITY: PRACTISING HOLDING BOUNDARIES OF CONFIDENTIALITY

Ask a colleague to question you as if they were the parent/carer of your young client, as follows:

- 'How is s/he getting on in counselling?'
- 'I am really worried about her/his bad behaviour at home; how does s/he behave with you?'
- 'How many more times do I need to bring her/him? S/he seems better to me.'
- 'Could you ask her/him how s/he feels about the new baby? S/he won't talk to me about it.'
- 'What's your secret? S/he seems to like you and hate me at the moment.'

Notice if you get tongue-tied or too defensive. Notice if you give too much information. You need to practise this before it happens.

Always talk to your supervisor if you feel you have said too much to a parent/carer/teacher or other adult involved with your client. The great majority of situations are redeemable, but prevention is far better than having to sort out a situation where you have disclosed too much. It can be damaging to the therapeutic alliance if a young client thinks you are talking with the other adults in their life about them, so be clear about what you will and won't say and stick to that.

All counsellors of children and young people need to understand the relevant laws and the legal framework in which they are counselling, recognising that these are not static and knowledge needs to be updated regularly. There will be questions, challenges and even suspicions concerning the way you keep confidentiality. Be prepared for them.

THE LEGAL FRAMEWORK

The moment we enter into counselling with a child or young person, we need to know whether we can keep what they share with us confidential. It is not sensible or skilful to meet a challenging situation and then respond reactively. Counsellors need to be proactive in understanding the legal framework they are counselling within (Mitchels and Bond 2011).

If the legal framework has not been studied, it is easy to think that either the client is old enough to consent to counselling or they are not and that this is defined by their chronological age (Jenkins 2007).

During the counselling relationship, counsellors may have to decide whether the youngster is at risk. It is vital that the basis on which such a decision is made can be explained and, if necessary, defended.

The idea that such decisions are easy and can be based on absolute rules given to us from employers or professional organisations is soon dispelled. Knowing when a young person is competent to give informed consent to confidential counselling means assessing their competence to understand what it is they are consenting to. This means that there is often no absolute rule, no exact age and no universal rulebook to tell the counsellor whether their client can consent to counselling.

The context in which a counsellor works may have its own 'rules' about confidentiality – there may be agency rules or school policies. The current legal framework offers the possibility for many youngsters to receive confidential counselling before they become adults at age 18. The counsellor's ability to offer this confidential counselling to young people is based on their right to be included in matters that directly affect them and on the 'Gillick' case decision.

It is important for those counselling children and young people to understand what 'Gillick competence' means and where the term comes from. Before investigating the origins of the term 'Gillick competence', consider the following case example.

> ## CASE EXAMPLE: A 13-YEAR-OLD REQUESTS CONFIDENTIAL COUNSELLING
>
> Jessie comes to see you in her lunch hour at school; she knocks on the door and asks if you can counsel her without her parents knowing. Her dad would never agree to her talking about 'family stuff' with a stranger, she says. She begins to describe the social and cultural background she comes from, and how her life is controlled and planned for her. She will study certain subjects that her parents decide on and then leave school as soon as possible to get married to a person who her parents agree is 'right'. She will not work after marriage and will be expected to have children in her late teens or early twenties. She makes the comment: 'My dad would kill me if he knew I was telling you this.' She then says she
>
> *(Continued)*

(Continued)

loves her mum and dad and doesn't want to be a bad and troublesome daughter. She is in top sets at school and loves art. She wants to go to college and study until she is at least 21 before settling down and having a family. Jessie looks you straight in the eye as she tells you this – she is upset at the idea of doing something her parents would disapprove of, but she is calm and considered about her own life choices. She then asks you if you can counsel her without her parents knowing.

Will you offer Jessie confidential counselling? Take account of the following:

- Some adults hold the view that a child of 13 is the responsibility of her parents and that, consequently, they need to know who she is talking to and what the subjects under discussion are.
- Others may believe that parents are 'wrong' to control a child so strictly and that the child must have a way to talk about what is happening to them in their life circumstances.
- The school where the counsellor is seeing Jessie may have a policy about parental involvement.
- Finally, there are Jessie's own wishes and her clear reasons for requesting her parents are not informed about her attendance at counselling.

So what can be offered to Jessie? If she is offered confidential counselling, the decision will be based on the 'Gillick principle'.

GILLICK COMPETENCE

Victoria Gillick asked her local health authority to assure her that none of her five daughters would be offered contraceptive advice or treatment under the age of 16. She lost her case – it was decided that the children could choose whether or not they took part in sex education, if they were of sufficient maturity to know what they were agreeing to. The resulting legal decision allows for children and young people who are competent to consent to confidential advice and counselling independent of their parents' wishes or consent. The general principles of the Gillick decision have been upheld through later challenges to it, with some modifications in the case of life-threatening situations.

Counsellors are not usually legal experts. A working knowledge of the Gillick case and the subsequent term 'Gillick competence' is, however, necessary when offering a confidential counselling service to young people. Younger children are not affected by the ruling as they would probably not be able to give informed consent – in this case, permission by an adult with parental responsibility is required. But what do we mean by 'younger children' in this context? The Children's Legal Centre (1997) offers us the clarification that 'It is unlikely that a child under 13 would be considered competent to consent'. Children aged under 13, particularly some 11- and 12-year-olds, may understand exactly what they are saying if, like Jessie in the case study above, they ask for confidential counselling.

Here, then, is the basis for offering Jessie confidential counselling. Can a slightly younger child than Jessie with good, coherent reasons be offered counselling without parental or guardian consent? Before examining this further, it is important to remind ourselves that the context in which the counselling is taking place will have a bearing on whether confidentiality can be offered. There are sometimes strong opinions and interpretations concerning confidential counselling for children and young people. The differences can be based on how we view children's rights.

These questions can be asked of yourself and others you know. Ask different age groups these questions. Asking a variety of cultural backgrounds may also offer the opportunity to consider a range of replies:

- Is a child or young person completely subject to the will of their parents/guardians until they reach 18?

- Does a child or young person have a right to a view or opinion on matters that directly affect them?

- Can a child or young person make choices completely independently of their parents/guardians?

The questions above (adapted from Jenkins 2013) can be seen to directly influence the way a counsellor would consider Jessie's request for confidential counselling. Jessie gave a description of her parents that led the counsellor to believe that her parents consider her to be subject to their will throughout her childhood. There is a basis to challenge this under the United Nations Convention on the Rights of the Child (UNICEF 1989), Article 12 of which refers to the 'right of the child to express an opinion and have that opinion taken into account, in any matter or procedure affecting the child'.

Here, again, it is possible that counsellors will need to step outside what might be considered the central, relational ground of counselling into the realms of accurate interpretation of the law. In order to do so skilfully, useful legal knowledge includes:

- the Gillick decision

- the United Nations Rights of the Child (UNICEF 1989)

- the Children's Act 1989 which offers statutory rights to all children.

Interpreting Gillick competence is a matter that requires us to make our own assessment. Counsellors working with children and young people will have to make their own decision about the ability of a child to competently consent when it is very likely that those with parental responsibility would object, as in the case of 'Jessie'.

It is not enough to say, if questioned, that confidentiality was kept because Jessie wanted it that way and she was not in danger. It is necessary for counsellors to understand the applicable legal framework, recognising that this legal framework changes as amendments are made to laws and statutes.

Daniels and Jenkins (2010: 20) offer insight and clarification for the therapist, explaining that 'it can be seen that counsellors and therapists have to make their own decisions about a child's level of maturity and understanding'. They go on to say that though the Gillick decision 'opens the door' to independent therapeutic work, the process of judging the child's level of understanding and their ability to give informed consent remains a problematic judgement for therapists to make. This can be anxiety provoking for the practitioner who needs to make an informed choice on a case-by-case basis, rather than being presented with the 'rule' to follow.

The 'Fraser Guidelines' (Gillick *v.* West Norfolk AHA 1985) offer help in deciding whether confidentiality can be maintained with a client. Lord Fraser re-examined the Gillick case and although the outcome was described in the case of a doctor's response to a girl asking for contraceptive advice, the points made are directly relevant to counselling and can be applied to the decision to offer a young person confidential counselling.

Competence to give consent can be tested by being able to answer 'yes' to the following statements, adapted from Lord Fraser's clarification of the Gillick decision:

- The young person understands what counselling is.
- A request is made for the young person to inform their parents and reasons have been given for not wanting this to happen.
- The young person's mental health may suffer if counselling is not undertaken.
- The best interests of the young person are served by the counselling going ahead without parental consent.
- The support system of the young person and the level of risk have been considered.
- The counsellor has consulted or will consult with their supervisor about the case.
- The client is of an age and a maturity to understand what consent to counselling means.

It is very likely that Jessie's case will meet all the conditions for counselling to go ahead. We need to recognise, however, that this action has potential consequences.

CASE EXAMPLE: JESSIE CONTINUED ... SHE TELLS HER PARENTS SHE HAS BEEN TO COUNSELLING

Later in the year, Jessie decides she is taking Art and not Geography in her options for year 11 exams. Her parents need to sign her 'options' form. Jessie gets cross when her parents refuse to sign until she changes to Geography instead of Art. Jessie then tells her parents, in the heat of an argument: 'the counsellor thinks I am very good at art and need to express myself'. Jessie's parents ask her some questions and discover that she has been counselled without their knowledge or consent. As this happened in Jessie's school, the designated member of the school staff (often known to the counsellor as the 'link' person) comes to the counsellor and says that Jessie's parents are unhappy about the counselling and don't understand why they were not consulted in the first place. At this point, the counsellor needs to be accountable for the decision to counsel Jessie. As a young client shows courage in participating in their own life choices, counsellors may need to be resilient when their practice and choices are questioned.

> If the level of reflective, thoughtful practice needed has been undertaken and the legal framework of the counselling properly considered, as well as the matter being discussed in supervision, then it will be easier for the counsellor to explain why Jessie has received confidential counselling.
>
> Both Jessie's parents and the counsellor believe they have acted in the best interests of Jessie. Jessie herself should have a say in what happens next. Sometimes the road can be 'bumpy' in these cases and the outcomes are not always what we hope for. It may be that the school head overrides Jessie's legal rights and says counselling cannot continue now that her parents have objected. Counsellors need to maintain best, ethical practice each step along the way and make sure they have consulted on cases like Jessie's. There is firm ground to stand on if a complaint is made. Sometimes, but far from always, a young person's own voice will be heard in these circumstances. The fact that the law and children's rights show that Jessie's wishes should be considered in a case like this does not means that it will happen in practice.
>
> When there are conflicts of interest like this, the counsellor may feel nervous, concerned, angry or unhappy about what is happening to Jessie. It is very important to remain calm and considered in approach when your professional judgement to hold confidentiality is questioned.

Skills of remaining calm when your judgement to keep confidentiality is challenged

When the moment comes that someone questions your reasons for offering confidential counselling, then remaining calm and taking a professional approach are crucial skills.

Preparation for the moment requires familiarity and an in-depth understanding of what has been outlined above. Broad statements like 'I think it is OK for me to counsel Jessie; she is probably competent' will arouse suspicion that you don't actually know what you are doing. A better statement is one such as: 'I have consulted my supervisor, considered the legal framework and I can explain why I am counselling Jessie confidentially'. The informed decision has been made that she is competent to consent on her own behalf to confidential counselling. If she did disclose anything to me that meant she was at risk of significant harm, I would take appropriate action to ensure her safety.'

To recap the steps that have led you to the decision to offer Jessie confidential counselling, you will have:

- consulted your supervisor, who is experienced in counselling children and young people
- understood your reasons for keeping confidentiality and how you differ in your approach from other professionals such as social workers and teachers
- considered the current legal framework in which you are counselling, including having knowledge of:
  o the 1989 Children's Act
  o the UN Rights of the Child (UNICEF 1989)

- o the decision in the 'Gillick' case
- o the Fraser guidelines

- ◆ studied specific guidelines for your country (Wales, Scotland and Northern Ireland differ in certain aspects from English law, e.g. there are children's rights from the Children's Commissioner in Wales that do not apply in England)
- ◆ read and practised applying the BACP Ethical Framework with particular emphasis on applying competing principles to ethical dilemmas – this includes having confidence in using such terms as 'beneficence' and 'autonomy' (see Chapter 6)
- ◆ become familiar with and received training on the child protection procedures that exist within the context you are counselling (see Chapter 6)
- ◆ clear, accessible contact procedures within the context of your workplace, knowing who to contact in urgent situations, whether it is the parent/carer of your client, the link person in a school or the manager of the agency employing you
- ◆ taken care of yourself, including taking appropriate breaks and having good support networks, both professional and personal
- ◆ recognised the legal framework on which decisions are made to gain the confidence to hold confidentiality as the basis for counselling to take place.

Hold in mind that if there are cases where disclosure must happen, it will be because of the level of risk the young client is experiencing. Confidentiality is rarely absolute and a young person should not be offered the illusion of complete, total confidentiality. An agreement or 'contract' that is fit for purpose will outline limits to a confidential counselling relationship.

There needs to be an agreement that is understood by the client. This agreement can be verbal or written. In either case, it should be tailored to meet the age and ability of the young client.

AGREEMENTS AND CONTRACTS

Counselling relationships with children and young people need to have an agreement or contract in place. If you are the type of counsellor that talks to young people on a sofa in a youth club, you still need to explain the basis on which you are offering counselling. A counsellor never knows what is going to be said to them. If a child or young person discloses something to you that you cannot keep confidential and you haven't explained how confidentiality works, you are doing them a great disservice. Transparency and honesty about what you can and cannot offer in terms of confidentiality are vital. Make sure you know the limits to confidentiality within the particular context you are counselling.

You may be the first counsellor a youth club or community group has ever had. It's up to you to both ask about and explain confidentiality.

CASE EXAMPLE: THE VOLUNTARY COUNSELLOR IN A NEW COMMUNITY CENTRE

You have been a counsellor for 10 years it is your second career which you began after your children left home. You work one day a week as a voluntary counsellor in a bereavement service. A friend from a neighbouring village asks you if you will come to their community centre's youth section and counsel some of the young people there. You are keen to help out and say that you will give it a try.

Here are some of the confidentiality and professional issues you need to consider:

- A quiet, private room is required for confidential counselling; is there one available? Many youth centres do not have such a room available and may think it will be acceptable for you to sit in a quiet corner. This is OK if you are a mentor or youth worker using counselling skills. If you want to offer counselling with an agreement to explore personal issues deeply, then a room is required. The room needs to be warm enough and have comfortable chairs and non-invasive décor. There should be no adverts for other activities such as religious services or workshops, practitioners, etc. in the room. When young people open up in counselling, they are making themselves vulnerable and a neutral space is best.

- A counsellor needs to have someone else on the premises whilst they are counselling. For safety reasons, being alone in a building with your client is not good practice. It could be a caretaker or a volunteer who is willing to chaperone. Ideally, it will not be the child or young person's parent/carer who takes this role, but if a client is seen for counselling outside of the usual hours that the community group meets, the parent/carer waiting in another room may be the best solution available.

- You need to have a written agreement and a meeting with the committee who run the community centre explaining how the counselling will be conducted. Check that the correct insurances are in place. It will probably be the case that children of committee members attend the youth group and they need to understand the confidential nature of counselling and the limits to confidentiality. People tend to be happy about the idea of confidential counselling until an issue arises that they are not expecting – you are counselling their 14-year-old daughter who they are concerned about, for example.

- Prepare the agreement you are going to make with your young clients. You need to have an agreement in place when you meet with your first client at the start of counselling. It's not acceptable to explain to a young client why you need to make a disclosure if they believed the counselling to be 100% confidential at the beginning.

- Be sure that your supervisor has clinical experience with children and young people (there is more on this in Chapter 8).

- Know who you will disclose to and how you will do so if the need arises.

(Continued)

> *(Continued)*
>
> - Remember that notes you write could be read by your client or used in a court of law (Data Protection Act). Keep your notes concise and factual. Be sure to keep them in a safe and secure manner.
> - If you and the community group want to go ahead with confidential counselling and can meet the conditions necessary, consider what is good practice in making an agreement with children and young people.

Good practice and pitfalls in making confidential counselling agreements

- First and foremost, do not offer absolute confidentiality.
- Never say 'It's our secret' or 'If you tell me what is bothering you so much, I will keep it to myself'.
- Explain all the terms you use. Avoid counselling jargon. Consider at what age you think most children understand the word 'confidentiality'.
- Do say to a younger client: 'I won't tell anyone what we talk about unless you are in danger of being hurt/harmed'. Explain to the parents/carers of a child who is not competent to consent to counselling that the subject matter of the sessions is private, as long as there are no risks to the child's safety.
- Identify to your client who it is that you are not going to talk to, e.g. 'I won't talk to your parents, teachers, friends or other family members about what we say unless you are at risk of being harmed and I need to help keep you safe'.
- Remember that for some children talking of possible 'harm' is confusing and potentially upsetting. An 11-year-old once gave me a detailed explanation of how he had grazed his knee after reading the question on an assessment form: 'have you ever thought of harming yourself?' Some children of this age do not know what self-harm is and have been fortunate enough not to have been harmed by others. They may have come to counselling due to a bereavement or difficult transition to a new school. It is a very delicate matter to explain the agreement without bringing in new ideas that may be inappropriate for young clients.
- Reassure your young client that if the confidentiality of the counselling needs to be broken, except in emergencies you will not disclose anything until you have told them you are going to do so and you will do your best to speak with them first about what is going to be said and to whom. Children and young people may sometimes want their counsellor to pass on something to the relevant adult.
- Do say to your young client that sometimes, but not very often, you need to tell others what has been said even if they don't want this. This will only happen if they are at risk of harm, but they may not agree that they are at risk or believe the risk is more manageable than it seems to the counsellor.

- Remember that the agreement must reflect the possibility that it will not always be the young client's view of the situation that prevails. A child or young person who is being abused can express love or loyalty towards the abusive person. They may have grown to believe that beatings are a normal part of life or that sexual behaviour toward them is their own fault and that somehow they 'made' their abuser behave that way. Counsellors must never be drawn into the secrecy of abusive behaviour. Children can hold beliefs such as that continuing to suffer abuse is better than a family member going to prison. This is understandable, but the child does not fully comprehend the consequences of the choice they are making. They may be conditioned or forced to comply with illegal and immoral acts. As counsellors, we must look in two directions at once on these occasions – deeply empathising with the plight of a child who cares for people who are mistreating them, whilst recognising that there may be a need to take immediate action where abuse is ongoing in a child's life. How to act is explained in more detail in the section on child protection (Chapter 6). Here, the focus is on the agreement or contract we are making, which needs to reflect the possibility of acting contrary to the child or young person's wishes in cases of abuse.

- Remember that a young client may genuinely fear for their safety if they 'tell'. A calm yet confident explanation of the limits to confidentiality should help to build the relationship and offer clarity about limits and boundaries.

- Remember when making your agreement that a child's level of development may prevent understanding of the consequences of their own behaviour. Very high levels of risk-taking behaviour can be viewed as fun – playing on railway lines or sniffing glue with friends, for example. Examples of this can be spoken about with young clients. Make sure explanations are tailored to the developmental age and competencies of the young client. Even the most difficult subjects can be framed in a positive way: 'It's part of my job to make sure that you are safe and if I think you are in danger, I might have to tell someone else because I only see you once a week.'

- Explain that you are not a friend, though you will be friendly, and in the end you are an adult with responsibilities.

When you were asked by your friend to take up a voluntary position as counsellor to young people in a community setting, there may not have been an awareness of all that is involved in doing so. Conditions must be met in order for safe and ethical counselling to take place.

In the next chapter, we will consider the ethics of practice with children and young people and how these interact with child protection procedures.

CHAPTER SUMMARY

- Confidentiality with children and young people is significantly different to confidentiality with adults in counselling.

- Young people can be offered confidential counselling without parental consent if they are competent to give informed consent to that counselling.

- The decision as to whether a young person is competent to consent to confidential counselling is based on whether they are 'Gillick' competent. It is necessary for counsellors to understand this case law and the 'Fraser guidelines' that followed from it.

- The context of the counselling will influence the counsellor's ability to keep confidentiality.

- Confidentiality is not absolute. The limits to confidentiality must be explained clearly.

- Disclosures need to be considered and carefully made to the right professional or agency where there is abuse or neglect happening in a child or young person's life. More on dilemmas and good practice concerning this follow in the next chapter.

- Make sure you know the correct procedure within your context for making a disclosure. Consult your supervisor and be prepared to find disclosure difficult. Don't rush to disclose to relieve your anxiety; often there are no easy answers and cause for concern is not always a reason to disclose. Young clients may not agree with your assessment of risk. In some cases, a disclosure needs to be made against a client's wishes (see Chapter 6).

- Keep the young client and the therapeutic alliance at the centre of your thoughts, feelings and actions. You are not counselling in isolation and all the professional issues raised here need to be considered thoroughly as a counsellor with children and young people.

REFERENCES

BACP/Welsh Assembly Government (WAG) (undated) *Schools Based Counselling Operating ToolKit*. Available at: www.bacp.co.uk/crs/Ethics%20in%20Practice/schoolToolkit.php

Bond, T.N. and Mitchels, B. (2008) *Confidentiality and Record Keeping in Counselling and Psychotherapy*. London: Sage.

Children's Legal Centre (1997) 'Offering children confidentiality: law and guidance', *Childright*, 142: 1–8.

Daniels, D. and Jenkins, P. (2010) *Therapy with Children: Children's Rights, Confidentiality and the Law*. London: Sage.

Department of Health (DoH) (1991) *The Children's Act 1989*. London: HMSO.

Gillick v. West Norfolk AHA (1985) Lord Fraser at 413.

Jenkins, P. (2007) *Counselling, Psychotherapy and the Law*. London: Sage.

Jenkins, P. (2013) *Children's Rights and Counselling*. Hove: Pavilion.

HBO (2012) *In Treatment*. DVD. Warner Home Video.

Mitchels, B. and Bond, T.N. (2011) *Legal Issues Across Counselling and Psychotherapy Settings: A Guide for Practice*. London: Sage.

UNICEF (1989) *UN Convention on the Rights of the Child*. London: Children's Rights Development Unit.

6

SKILLS FOR RESOLVING ETHICAL DILEMMAS

INTRODUCTION

This chapter aims to equip and support counsellors with a variety of skills to make an informed ethical decision.

Situations arise that do not have a single right answer, and these can cause anxiety. Counsellors need to embrace this, knowing that there is no one path that can completely satisfy everyone when there are competing ideologies and views. Courage and up-to-date knowledge are prerequisites when resolving ethical dilemmas, as are a sense of balance, self-awareness and professional competence.

We will discover the qualities that blend together to create a flexible, warm-hearted, committed approach when faced with the heat and pressure of ethical dilemmas. Those dilemmas that arise frequently are explored, with the recognition that there are no easy solutions to them. Counsellors need skills and composure when faced with challenging and potentially distressing problems.

The ethical dilemmas chosen for this chapter aim to address current concerns of counsellors with children and young people:

- dilemmas that arise from social, online and mobile forms of media and communication
- child protection issues and how to manage a 'cause for concern' that may or may not require a disclosure
- issues around confidentiality, linking with the previous chapter.

In this chapter, we will look at:

- applying the BACP Ethical Framework and 'Competing Principles' to address ethical dilemmas
- a model for ethical decision making, with exercises and application to counselling children and young people

- making ethical choices
- child protection issues
- client confidentially with new technologies including texting, mobiles and social networking
- the context of counselling
- liaising with others in the 'helping professions'
- counsellors attending multi-agency meetings
- specific issues for school counselling
- self-care and mindful approaches to ethical practice.

> **MINDFUL MOMENT: YOUR ETHICAL SELF**
>
> Breathe in and out evenly, take a moment to relax your body and perhaps have a mindful tea break.
> Consider what it means for you to be involved in a dilemma where there is no one right answer. Do you enjoy the challenge? Do you want someone else to decide for you? Are you determined to fight for what you believe is right? Can you be defensive and cross? Whatever your particular way is when faced with a dilemma, take the time to get to know it a little better. As best you can, bring calm awareness to your journey with any dilemma. Know that you will do the best you can and that you are able to return to just breathing for a moment at any stage along the way.

APPLYING THE BACP ETHICAL FRAMEWORK

The BACP Ethical Framework asks counsellors to engage in 'ethical mindfulness' (Gabriel and Casemore 2010) – there are no prescriptive rules; rather, we decide on the best course of action, taking into account the obligation to provide adequate care for our clients.

Counsellors can find the terminology in the Ethical Framework difficult at first. It is worth becoming familiar with the language used. Within some unfamiliar terms are very helpful ideas that help in ethical decision making.

The moral principles in the BACP Ethical Framework are:

- being trustworthy (fidelity)
- autonomy
- beneficence
- non-maleficence

- justice
- self-respect.

Examples follow of how each of the above principles is relevant when counselling children and young people.

Being trustworthy (fidelity)

Being trustworthy asks that we keep in mind the importance of trust in the counsellor/client relationship. It reminds us that we need to be trustworthy when counselling children and young people. The principle of being trustworthy is frequently challenged when the client is a child. A young client speaks to us about their private life, and they do so believing they can trust us with their deepest feelings, most worrying thoughts and challenging circumstances. We need to be worthy of this trust by explaining carefully what we can and cannot keep confidential (see Chapter 5) and then honouring trust by remaining within the boundaries of the confidential relationship.

Motives for being trustworthy in holding confidentiality with a child or young person can be misunderstood by other professionals, parents and carers.

Skills of being trustworthy

Attending a multi-agency meeting When asked to share information about a young client in a multi-agency meeting, there can initially be confusion or shock when we explain that we need to maintain confidentiality of the counselling relationship. Think of 'being trustworthy' as the moral principle that we are upholding at these times. This can help to de-personalise any potential conflict. It is not our personal opinion or need, but our professional role of being trustworthy in holding the confidences of clients that is in action.

Holding the principle of being trustworthy or of fidelity clearly in mind when asked to speak about our young client's issues to others will help to maintain the appropriate boundaries of the confidential counselling relationship. A child or young person has trusted us; we then act 'in accordance with the trust' (BACP 2013) placed in us. This principle needs to be balanced with consideration of the other principles to make the best decision possible.

Counsellors also need to consider being trustworthy in everyday life. Being trustworthy ideally needs to be part of us, not a cloak we put on in the counselling role. Most counsellors will be trustworthy much of the time, and working towards upholding any moral principle is a journey and requires a great deal of reflection.

Summary of skills in being trustworthy:

- Maintain boundaries of confidentiality.
- Reflect on choices.
- Use mindfulness in everyday life.

Autonomy

The principle of autonomy features as a major issue when clients are children or young people. In counselling adults, questions of autonomy arise occasionally. With young clients, autonomy or lack of it is often a central theme. Autonomy is defined as: 'respect for the client's right to be self-governing' (BACP 2013: 2). As discussed in the previous chapter, children and young people have limited rights to be self-governing. In many instances, particularly if they are aged 11–12 or under, children may not be allowed to come to counselling without the consent of an adult with parental responsibility. The definition of autonomy needs to be re-considered when the client is a child.

Skills of autonomy

Counselling is voluntary It is a regular occurrence that children arrive in the counselling room having very little idea of why they are there and even less knowledge of what counselling is. It is incumbent upon the counsellor to explain the nature of counselling and discover whether the young client has at least a wish to try it and see what it's like. Autonomy is very important for children and young people in counselling, though there is a need to recognise that there are differences in the autonomy of a child from that of an adult. We may need to explain to adults who want their child to come to counselling why that child needs to agree to attend. The voluntary nature of counselling applies to the young as much as anyone else.

Within the counselling relationship, respecting a young client's autonomy may mean recognising that their views differ from those of their parents or teachers, and never becoming a 'mouthpiece' for adults who are trying to persuade them to change.

Summary of skills in autonomy:

- Act in accordance with children's rights.
- Respect your client's view.
- Encourage your client to be appropriately self-governing according to their age and circumstances.

Beneficence

Beneficence means having a commitment to promote the client's well-being. In the BACP Ethical Framework, it states: 'An obligation to act in the best interests of a client may become paramount when working with clients whose capacity for autonomy is diminished because of immaturity' (BACP 2013: 2).

This clearly has relevance for those counselling children and young people. What is suggested here is that the principle of beneficence will need to be given more weight, and it 'may become paramount' to act on behalf of a young client.

The need to act in the best interests of a young client also shows the importance of having a supervisor who is experienced with issues concerning children and young people in counselling. It is all too easy to miss a vital moment where we need to act on behalf of our client, wrongly presuming procedures are the same as when clients are adults.

Skills of beneficence

Unintended consequences A child may hold loyalty to an abusive or neglectful parent or be taking part in extremely risky behaviour. There are consequences of this that are unforeseen by the client due to their young age and limited life experience. A young client saying they are happy with their life will not be enough of a reason for the counsellor to hold confidentiality where there is current, ongoing abuse or neglect. After due thought and consultation (this may have to take place very quickly), the counsellor will act in a beneficent manner in the client's best interests. This means informing social services and the police who can act to protect a young client, even if the client themselves does not want this to happen. The young client needs to be informed of actions taken on their behalf and supported throughout the process of disclosure.

Sometimes we are not sure whether our client is in danger or not. Disclosures happen over time and are often not clearly stated at first. As we shall find later in the chapter, this is where ethical dilemmas arise. Having a clear understanding of the principle of beneficence is an important 'building block' in the process of making the best ethical choice possible.

Summary of skills in beneficence:

- Recognise unintended consequences.
- Consult with your supervisor and other professionals where necessary.
- Support clients throughout each stage of any disclosure.

Non-maleficence

Children and young people in counselling are vulnerable and it is vital to avoid harming them. It's a hefty responsibility to be alone in a room with a child, the door shut and keeping their confidences. For many young clients, this may be a unique experience. Within the principle of non-maleficence, counsellors are expected to mitigate any harm 'even when the harm is unavoidable or unintended' (BACP 2013: 2). We must be careful not to promise children or young people anything that we cannot carry through.

Sometimes counsellors act in harmful ways towards young clients unintentionally. Examples of this include giving money to them or counselling in rooms where there is no possibility of confidentiality.

Skills in non-maleficence

Money and gifts Giving money or gifts to children and young people can appear to be an act of kindness, particularly if a child is clearly hungry or does not have enough clothes. It is problematic to ignore symptoms of excessive hunger and neglect in a child and counsellors should not do so. Compassionate action needs to be taken if a child is cold, hungry or terrified. The action may need to be indirect, via a pastoral member of staff in a school, for example, in order to maintain a counselling rather than a welfare role. It may be possible to donate to a school fund that will be used to help children such as your client, if you want to help. Giving money directly to your client can create both dependency and secrets. It may be important to raise concerns about a child's welfare – if they have no money for lunch, for example, this can be done without breaking the confidential relationship. You may need to advocate for the child, with their agreement and permission on a practical matter. This is preferable to privately giving money or gifts, as doing so is likely to cause unintended harm and possibly dependency.

Privacy of counselling rooms Counselling young clients should not take place in rooms where people walk in without knocking, such as other people's offices or in jointly used spaces or partitioned rooms with paper-thin walls where everything can be overheard. We need to uphold the principle of privacy when counselling children and young people in order to be non-maleficent. Counsellors sometimes say 'the client doesn't mind being identified or interrupted'. Young clients in their first experience of counselling have no idea what to expect. It is up to you as their counsellor to avoid harming them by protecting the confidential nature of counselling and making sure they have privacy. Clear notices on doors and an insistence that it is not acceptable to be interrupted are part of upholding this principle (McGinnis with Jenkins 2006).

Summary of skills in non-maleficence:

- Act compassionately and ethically to ensure clients have basics such as food and clothing.
- Protect confidentiality of rooms where counselling takes place.
- Question and consult on your own actions to avoid unintended harm.

Justice

Children and young people have a very strong sense of justice. They will tell you it's 'not fair' that others can do things that they are forbidden to do. For counsellors, holding the principle of justice can be challenging. This principle asks us to 'remain alert to potential conflicts between legal and ethical obligations' (BACP 2013: 2). When child protection issues are discussed later in the chapter, it will be seen that law is not always the same as justice. This principle also asks us to 'be committed to equality of opportunity' (BACP 2013: 2).

Skills of justice

Siblings in school A school counsellor can be working with siblings without initially realising that this is the case. If two clients have a surname that is shared by many, there is no way to know if they are closely related until the counselling has become well established. If two siblings do not know the other is coming to counselling, what is the 'just' way for the counsellor to proceed in this case once s/he finds out they are siblings? Often, there is one counsellor at a school, so not continuing counselling with both of them means that one is denied access to counselling and does not have equality of opportunity to receive the service. The counsellor will need to do their best to make sure their individual confidentiality is maintained. If the counsellor does continue with both siblings, then the principle of justice asks us to keep their cases separate and minimise how one case influences the other. A supervisor's help is needed to manage this situation.

Other issues We also need to be aware of the position of young clients who do not share our first language. Do we need to consider interpreters or is this too much of an intrusion into the privacy of counselling?

Questions need to be asked concerning whether the counselling room is accessible to wheelchair users and whether those children and young people with a diagnosed condition such as ADHD or Autism can make use of counselling.

Justice requires that such issues are considered deeply and that we offer 'fair and impartial treatment' and 'adequate services' to all clients.

Summary of skills in justice:

- Challenge any lack of equality of opportunity in your counselling environment.
- Develop fluency with issues of diversity.
- Enable all potential clients to access counselling.

Self-respect

Without self-respect, the principles of the Ethical Framework cannot be put into practice. Counsellors develop as practitioners by applying all the ethical principles as 'entitlements for self'. This is particularly relevant when managing ethical dilemmas. The more deeply embedded the principle of self-respect is in the person of the counsellor, the more personal resources will be available when difficult and challenging situations arise.

Young people value the concept of respect very highly – often they are asked to respect others but do not feel they are respected in return. Mutual respect is a key concept when counselling children and young people. Introducing the idea of self-respect to young clients once we have embraced it ourselves can be very helpful. The crucial matter here is not to leave ourselves out, asking or expecting something of others that we don't practise in our own lives. We need to know ourselves well in order to be good enough counsellors.

Summary of skills in self-respect:

- Know your own strengths and limitations.
- Act in accordance with 'mutual respect'.
- Take care of yourself, recognising your own needs.

REFLECTIVE ACTIVITY: APPLYING THE BACP ETHICAL FRAMEWORK PRINCIPLES TO YOURSELF

- Write a short concise memo to yourself, a sentence that reminds you what each principle means to you, for example: Trustworthy means to me that I am reliable, I 'walk my talk'. Or non-maleficence means I won't hurt anyone and I will check out with others to make sure I'm not doing something wrong that I haven't noticed.

- Note the times in the last week when you have put these principles into action in your everyday life for yourself, in your family or at work.

- Describe the principles in simple language to a friend or family member, and ask them to give you feedback about your strengths and areas for development connected with these principles. Which of the ethical principles do you find you're good at applying? Which do you need to strengthen with your knowledge and ability? Perhaps you accept that you are a trustworthy person, regularly doing what you have said you will do in your everyday life. Can you, however, be too kind – too eager to act on behalf of someone, for example? Beneficence might be a very familiar action that needs to be balanced with more attention to your own autonomy, your ability to be self-governing.

- When you have chosen a principle to develop, ask a colleague or your supervisor to help you monitor progress towards greater embodiment of that principle. Remind yourself that you can probably use these principles already – it's just a question of refining and honing your abilities.

- Become familiar with the terminology of the principles and enjoy balancing them and considering how they 'compete'. If you are in a learning or supervision group, try to have each person embody a different principle. Discuss a current case in your own practice and see what each person offers as they speak with just that one principle in mind.

What are 'competing principles'?

Principles compete in the sense that they cannot always exist easily side by side. Offering young clients a private space to talk and being trustworthy within the counselling agreement (fidelity) may directly conflict at times with your duty to keep them safe from harm (non-maleficence). The fact that principles offer differing approaches to the same situation helps in understanding the complexities that exist in a dilemma.

Ethical decision making

Gabriel and Casemore (2010) offer a process model of ethical decision making. Often, the first thoughts when a dilemma arises are about what to do next. The model put forward asks the counsellor to consider their dilemma, asking whose problem it is and moving forward step by step. In their model: 'A dilemma is regarded … as a state of uncertainty or perplexity, especially requiring a choice between two equally unfavourable or favourable options where a choice must be made' (2010: 3).

Resolving ethical dilemmas

It is useful to have a method of working through ethical dilemmas step by step. Joyce and Sills (2014) offer a 12-point checklist that can be used as a framework to make sure all the important issues are covered. The framework is outlined below:

1. Summarise the dilemma.
2. Identify the ethical issues involved.
3. Find the section of your ethics code (e.g., the BACP Ethical Framework) that applies.
4. Identify the values that are in conflict.
5. Check any legal constraints.
6. Consider all possible options for action (or inaction).
7. Arrange consultation or supervision (before making a decision; see Chapter 8).
8. Assess the possible consequences of each decision you could make.
9. Choose the decision that would have the least damaging consequences or the best outcome overall.
10. Make a written record of your considerations and the recommendations of your supervisor (with dates).
11. Plan how to support yourself to live with the decision.
12. Take the action you have chosen.

(Adapted from Joyce and Sills 2014: 281)

Using this approach gives us the ability to tackle ethical dilemmas skilfully. Alongside these skills, it is necessary to understand how social services apply child protection guidelines to keep children and young people safe.

UNDERSTANDING CHILD PROTECTION

Child protection guidelines are based on principles that attempt to ensure children are 'free from abuse, victimisation and exploitation. Children should also be listened to, respected and have a safe home which supports physical and emotional well-being' (All Wales Child Protection Procedures 2008). Four types of abuse are identified: physical, emotional, sexual and neglect.

> The Children's Act 1989 introduced the concept of significant harm as the threshold that justifies intervention in family life in order to protect children. Significant harm is defined in the legislation as ill treatment or the impairment of health and development … There is no absolute criteria on which to rely when judging what constitutes significant harm. (All Wales Child Protection Procedures 2008: 59)

Counsellors with children and young people need to understand how child protection works; it is not the duty of the counsellor to decide if any particular case constitutes significant harm or not. The counsellor needs to decide in each case, in consultation with their supervisor, if there is sufficient cause for concern that social services must be informed so that the steps necessary to protect the child can be taken. Social services then decide whether there is significant harm taking place.

It is good practice for everyone involved with counselling children and young people to know who to contact should the need arise. A cause for concern can occur suddenly and unexpectedly. Being prepared leads to more ease in managing ethical and professional decision making.

Counsellors who have made child protection referrals will recognise that what happens next is variable. Social services departments are busy and they have their own professional procedures that are different from those of counsellors. Sometimes after a child protection referral by a counsellor, there is a big investigation involving police, searches and arrests. Sometimes very little happens – there is a call to the home of the client by a social worker, a short chat with the child and the case is closed. Often, the counsellor is not involved in this process at all. There may be a discrepancy between the counsellor's assessment of need for intervention and that of social services. Counsellors may want either more involvement or less action taken on behalf of their young client, depending on what has been disclosed.

When a young client is clearly in need of social services and wants this help, the counsellor can take the role of a figure who maintains regular contact through a time of change. It is usually, but not always, when the client does not want a disclosure to take place that dilemmas arise in counselling.

Daniels and Jenkins (2010) ask us to consider the following when deciding whether to report abuse. Counsellors may decide against an automatic reporting response where:

- the abuse is historic rather than current
- the young person strongly opposes disclosure (Gillick principle)
- the abuse is not immediately life-threatening

- other children are not at risk from the same abuse
- other professionals are currently monitoring the young client
- the young client is aware of other potential sources of help.

Recently, there has been a challenge to the discretion of those working with children being able to hold confidentiality when abuse is disclosed. Online petitions have asked that we support mandatory reporting of suspected child abuse in order to protect children. It can seem difficult to explain how having discretion in when and how to report a child's abuse can be in their best interests. Some public figures with power and influence have now been confirmed as having been child abusers. Some of the abused, now adults, have spoken about their abusive experiences. When the abuse took place and they disclosed to adults, they were ignored or punished for their honesty. There is clearly a need for something to change – more children need to be protected from abuse and some believe mandatory reporting will help.

Mandatory reporting can deprive vulnerable young people of a safe space to talk confidentially. Informed and well-judged discretionary reporting is in the best interests of young clients. Counsellors do not want a child to remain in a dangerous or abusive situation. We need, though, to fully understand the position of the young client (Jenkins 2013). Disclosures happen over time, so we may have to decide whether there is a need to act on the young client's behalf (beneficence) or whether to respect their wishes (autonomy) and the privacy they have come to counselling for.

There has been an informed request by Professor Ashton, president of the Faculty of Public Health, to lower the age of ability to consent to sex from 16 to 15 years (Withnall 2013). This request has not been accepted by the government. Professor Ashton said that society had to accept that a third of young people aged 14 and 15 were having sex. Acts of under-age sex are considered to be child protection issues. This means that a third of young people are 'breaking the law' and having to hide their sexual activity. Lowering the age of consent could help young people aged 15, who feel ready to be sexual with a partner of a similar age, to stay on the right side of the law.

Deciding on the best possible ethical choice for young clients

You need:

1. Knowledge of relevant legislation and case law concerning confidentiality and child protection guidelines.
2. Familiarity with the BACP Ethical Framework, particularly the 'moral principles', considering how they compete (see above).
3. Understanding of ethical decision-making processes (outlined above).

4. Engagement in case-specific, up-to-date research, e.g. for a case involving self-harm, read 'Self-harm: the solution not the problem' (Martin 2013).

5. To hold in mind awareness of limitations on choices due to agency/employer contracts and the context of the counselling.

Developing a 'practical wisdom' (Owens et al. 2012) and holding the balance between safety and creativity is at the heart of effective ethical practice.

The following case examples raise ethical dilemmas about maintaining a confidential counselling relationship. Combine all the guidance given in this chapter when deciding how to act.

CASE EXAMPLES

1 Under-age sex

Sara attends the youth club where you counsel. She has just had her 15th birthday and tells you she is in a sexual relationship with Gary who is 22. Sara has been to her GP who has given her contraception. Gary lives locally and has a job and a car which appeals to Sara; Sara doesn't want anyone else to know about this. You recognise that, in law, Gary could be seen as abusing Sara. The sex is consensual in the sense that it is not forced, and Sara wants the sexual relationship. Sara, however, is not old enough to consent to sex. Some would consider this a matter that needed to be referred to the police. If mandatory reporting were operational, the counsellor would be required to report Sara's disclosure as a child protection issue. Whilst this is a cause for concern, Sara does not seem to be in danger. We need to be aware that sexual exploitation is a growing problem. There is no sign that Sara is being coerced or groomed, but, because of her age, we need to see her as vulnerable and inexperienced in such matters: could Sara be unaware of certain risks in her situation? Would you as her counsellor keep confidentiality with her in this circumstance?

2 Sexual abuse is suspected but not disclosed

Berta, aged 12, pops in to see you every so often at the school where you are a counsellor and repeatedly talks to you about a 'friend' who is being abused by her step-father, but who can't tell anyone because she would be breaking up the family. You have encouraged Berta to tell her friend to come to counselling, expressed this as a cause of concern to your supervisor and recently asked Berta directly if her friend is actually her and explained you cannot knowingly leave a child or young person in an abusive situation. Berta starts to back off rapidly – her friend was probably just talking about a story she saw on TV – it's nothing to worry about, she says. You feel that if you question her further at this stage she will not return to counselling. In your previous contact with social services, you have been involved with young people who have retracted disclosures of abuse and you know that the young person might be left in a more vulnerable and difficult life situation if this happens. Are there any further actions you would need to take at this time?

3 Signs of physical abuse

Jack is 10 and regularly comes to school with unusual bruises. His teachers are worried that he is being hit at home and he is sent to counselling. He has a bruise on the top of his head; he tells you how clumsy he is, always falling over. He says he doesn't really want counselling but he is happy to play cards with you and chat a bit. You notice that if you make a sudden movement he flinches. You gently draw attention to his jumpiness, just saying what you noticed. Jack looks at you, his eyes filling with tears, but after a brief moment his cheeky jokes return, he shrugs his shoulders and he continues with the card game. Would you pass on any concerns about Jack to others – if so, to whom?

4 Historical abuse and threats of violence

Antonio is 17 when he comes to see you in your private practice. His parents are paying for his sessions because they are concerned about angry outbursts where he has hit walls and doors at home. He stays in his bedroom, has contact with friends on social media and plays violent, adult electronic games for many hours each day. He has dropped his college course where he was studying music technology, tends only to get up in the late afternoon and uses his money for occasional binges of alcohol and 'a laugh' out with his friends. Antonio tells you about an episode in his past where he was sexually abused by his uncle. This happened 10 years ago and he has not told anyone in order to protect his mother. His uncle is now in prison for fraud so cannot currently be a danger to other children, he says. When his uncle is released from prison, Antonio plans to beat him up. You ask him if he understands that what he is proposing is illegal and explain that any action to take the law into his own hands might mean he would have a criminal record. He says it's the best way as far as he is concerned. Antonio says he is prepared to discuss his pent-up anger and think everything through. Do you need to act outside of the confidential relationship in this circumstance?

5 Self-harm

Rema comes to see you in the school where you counsel. She is 14 and has been diagnosed with a condition that gives her lots of pain in her body. She has to rest and needs to learn to relax and unwind as this helps her feel better. You have been seeing her for a few sessions when she tells you she is self-harming. She is very ashamed of this and particularly afraid that her younger siblings will find out about it and copy her behaviour, as they look up to her. She describes her family as being very caring, but there is a definite 'get on with it and don't

(Continued)

(Continued)

complain or fuss' attitude in her home life. You begin to talk with Rema about the self-harm – both of you know that there is a school policy of informing parents about children self-harming. Rema is adamant that no one must know. You talk together about the school's policy and safer ways to self-harm, and you ask her if she would be able to tell someone else – the school nurse, for example – as you only see her once a week. She says no because she can't trust them not to tell her parents. Eventually, she shows you the self-harm, and you feel quite relieved as there are just small scratches on her upper arms, no deep wounds. She tells you that this is the extent of her self-harm and you believe this to be the case. It's Rema's self-disgust, shame and guilt that concern you. You are aware though of the school's policy on self-harm. What is the best way to proceed in this case?

6 Ill health

Zahir, aged 14, comes to see you for counselling in the school where you counsel following a family bereavement. Everyone at home is sad, he says, and he feels invisible. He doesn't want to make a fuss about anything and he has been feeling that his medication for a serious health condition has made everything worse. He feels exhausted in the mornings and unable to concentrate. You make a note of his condition, which is unfamiliar to you, and of the name of the medication. You talk to him about discussing this problem with his parents or going to his GP or the school nurse. He doesn't want to take up any of these options. You decide to continue counselling him and check in with him about his medication. Three weeks later, when you ask him how he is doing on his medicine now, he tells you that he hasn't taken his meds for the past fortnight and actually feels better. You feel concerned that just stopping his prescribed medication might hold unknown risks for Zahir. You share your concerns with him. He gets a bit edgy and says he has come to talk to you about a death in his family, so can you 'drop it' about the meds. You feel concerned that raising the subject again will drive him out of counselling. You worry too that he might be storing up problems for himself by not taking his medicine. You decide to call a confidential helpline anonymously to try and get more information about his medical condition. You also plan to talk to your supervisor – all this takes time and you are not sure if you should disclose this to your 'link person' in the school straightaway. You know she would phone his parents and Zahir would feel betrayed by this action. What is the best course of action in this case?

7 Neglect and emotional abuse

Megan is 9; you have received lots of information about her before you meet her. Right now she is in foster care, whilst her mother is an addicted substance misuser and involved in criminal activity to maintain her addiction. Megan has been neglected. She often curls up in a foetal position in the counselling room; she is small, pale and thin. She is not allowed to have any contact with her mum

> at the moment, though there is a hope that this will change when her mum comes out of 'rehab'. Megan has a much older half-sister who comes to visit her regularly and takes her out to the park. Megan is drawing a picture and, almost by chance, starts to talk about being on the swings and her sister's phone ringing and 'guess what, it was my mum!' 'I talked to her for ages and she asked if I was OK', Megan tells you. She puts her finger on her lips and says 'my sister says it's a secret, I am not supposed to tell anyone'. She carries on with her drawing, singing to herself quietly. What do you do next in this situation?

Remember:

- Where younger children (those not Gillick competent) are involved, sharing information becomes more pressing and urgent. There are very good reasons to appropriately disclose to keep 'Jack' safe from physical abuse and 'Megan' safe in her foster placement. These two dilemmas are included as they involve disclosure when the child does not want this to happen.
- Each one of the above cases requires courage and a determination to put the young client's best interests at the heart of the decision making.
- Apply the processes given above (page 129) for resolving ethical dilemmas to each of the case studies, remembering there is often not a single right answer.

When a client wants us to intervene on their behalf

> ### CASE EXAMPLE: KIM WANTS HER INOCULATION
>
> Kim is 13 and wants to consent to an inoculation in school that her parents don't want her to have. She comes to see the school counsellor to ask for help to consent on her own behalf. The counsellor wants to help her and is aware that she has rights.
>
> #### The counsellor
>
> 'I have read the UN Rights of the Child and believe s/he is Gillick competent' (see Chapter 5). 'She should be able to consent herself to this inoculation.' The counsellor then asks a colleague who is a counsellor and a qualified paediatric nurse for an opinion.
>
> *(Continued)*

> *(Continued)*
>
> ### A counsellor who is also a paediatric nurse
>
> 'I have seen young people, 13, 14 and 15 years old, in great pain having broken bones, waiting for their parents to arrive at the hospital before consent for an operation to reset bones is given. Medics will often not accept consent from a young person. There is a fear of litigation. They won't give her the inoculation without parental consent.'
>
> ### The client's parents
>
> 'Of course, a young person of 13 doesn't understand what they are consenting to. If she reacts to the inoculation and becomes ill, we, her parents, will be involved so we need to have the final say about this.'
>
> ### The counsellor's supervisor
>
> Although the young person has expressed their concern in counselling about not having this inoculation, it is not within our remit to change the practices of other professions. We can encourage our client to believe that she has a right to her own opinion concerning her own body. There may be an appropriate referral to the school nurse or her GP to get advice about having the inoculation.

We expect other professionals to respect our practice; we also need to allow others to conduct themselves according to their guidelines. In the appropriate place – perhaps a meeting between professionals – we can raise concerns about young people's rights not being respected and their voices not being heard, but we may not be able to intervene.

If, however, we believe we have witnessed or heard a disclosure of abuse or neglect by an institution or other professional, as well as by a parent/carer, then we need to take action even if others try to dissuade us from doing so.

Kim's counsellor can maintain a counselling relationship with her and perhaps she will be able to get the inoculation she wants via her GP. Kim can talk with you about how she will live with her situation until she is considered old enough by the medical profession to give consent on her own behalf.

A counsellor's influence is limited outside of the counselling room and choosing to challenge other professionals must be done with great care. Good working relationships are vital but that doesn't mean colluding or keeping silent when something is seriously wrong. The necessity for school counsellors to be independent of other school staff and not be friends with them or seek their approval is highlighted here.

SCHOOL COUNSELLORS — INDEPENDENT OR PART OF A PASTORAL TEAM?

An ethical issue for counsellors in schools is how far they are independent of the school and how much they are part of the school 'team' of support workers and pastoral care. Different models of school counsellors have developed over time:

1. A teacher who trains and becomes a counsellor, integrating the two roles. The person in this role is very much a member of the school staff.

2. An independent counsellor, placed in a school with a designated 'link' person within the school with whom they liaise.

3. A counsellor employed by the school and part of the pastoral team.

Reasons for independence

As a result of the Clywch Report (2004), led by Peter Clarke, the First Children's Commissioner in Wales (a report into sexual abuse by a drama teacher), the following recommendation was made and acted upon by the Welsh Assembly:

> A National Strategy for the provision of an independent children's counselling service for children and young people in education including the provision of appropriate support to children during disciplinary, child protection, complaints and exclusion processes. (Clarke 2004: 21.29)

An independent counsellor is now in every secondary school in Wales and every child and young person aged 11–18 has a right to access counselling at school.

The independent counsellor within a school can:

- represent and form an alliance with a child without being overly influenced by the school staff's opinion or ideas about that child or young person

- notice if a number of serious problems with one particular teacher or situation are raised by young clients in counselling and act in a beneficent manner without jeopardising their position

- question referrals from teachers of children who are disruptive in class, when very well behaved children who may be troubled and experiencing problems at home are not referred and, in some cases, are unsure how to access the school counsellor

- offer advice and information to school staff as to what counselling is and is not and how best to refer potential clients to the counselling service; this may involve meetings with heads of year in the school

- encourage and develop a self-referral system to counselling in the school; attending a school assembly to give general information about counselling helps with this.

A dilemma arises for the school counsellor: they need to be independent *and* on good terms with school staff. They might feel isolated or misjudged as aloof.

Skills for school counsellors in remaining independent whilst maintaining good relationships with school staff:

- Be professional and remember your counselling role.
- Discourage gossip and snippets of information about clients given to you in corridors or the staffroom (see Chapter 5).
- Encourage links and discussions about the counselling service with youth workers, the school nurse, CAMHS representatives in the school and teachers with pastoral responsibility.
- Keep in contact with other school counsellors in the area and talk about any feelings of isolation with your supervisor.
- Never be tempted to give 'off the record' information about your client to school staff that breaks the confidentiality agreement.
- Don't automatically accept another's 'view' of your client or a situation that is contrary to your own experience.
- If a child protection disclosure is needed, know who to contact in the school and act in accordance with guidelines.

CHILDREN AND YOUNG PEOPLE ONLINE — ETHICAL PRACTICE AND SKILLS

We exist at a time of ever-changing, developing virtual and mobile technology. Computers and mobile phones are a part of our everyday lives. For most young clients, their knowledge of new technologies goes way beyond having a mobile phone. Many young people are highly able and 'savvy' in the virtual world. Some live their lives very publicly, sharing their 'status' on social media, negotiating chat rooms and playing games with others who they may never have met. Ethical issues arise in counselling because of young clients' experience online. Counselling young people online is also a growing field (see www.kouth.com).

We can usefully remember that we have a responsibility to take seriously and engage in a thoughtful relationship with the society in which we and our clients live. (Johns 2012). We cannot assume knowledge and understanding of the world our young clients exist within. Some counsellors will be familiar and comfortable in the virtual worlds that young people inhabit, whilst many others will not.

How do counsellors ethically communicate through new technology with young clients? What are the skills needed to respond to the life experience of children and young people in a technological revolution?

There is a variety of ways that counsellors can engage with their clients through technology, from reminding clients of appointments by text to playing virtual games with clients within the counselling process.

Using texts/mobile phone calendars for client appointments

Young clients have problems in their ability to remember an appointment. Younger children are brought to counselling by adults, and counsellors in schools have various reminders and methods to get young people to their appointments. In some contexts, however, asking a client if they would like a carefully worded text reminder that just says 'appt with me tomorrow at 10am', for example, or suggesting they put the appointment into their mobile phone is a good response to young people's style of communication.

Having a 'page' on social media sites

There are debates about whether counsellors should have a 'public profile' of any kind on social media. It is very difficult to maintain confidentiality in this world. A young client may try to contact their counsellor on a social media site. Ignoring them or refusing a request to be friends online may impact on the counselling relationship. Accepting young clients as friends is not ethical if it will give access to personal information about us and our family. Good boundaries are vital in the virtual world. We can explain boundaries of how we will and won't communicate with young clients as part of our initial agreement.

Contacting clients via email

Specialist training is now available for counsellors who wish to use email as a method of contact. Contracts need to be very clear as the whole of any communication via email can be publicised easily. Emails can be forwarded to many people at the click of a button.

Virtual technology and games in counselling

As part of the process of counselling with children and young people, we use play (see Chapter 7). Can we include online games via a tablet in this play? Young people who have difficulty in talking can show much more of themselves through a game they are familiar with and are able to play well. There are creative, non-violent online games.

Counsellors need to be experienced and comfortable with the technology before introducing it into the counselling room.

Dr Tanya Byron, in her report on children in the digital age (2008), explains how much children and young people enjoy and value new technologies: 'Overall, children and young people were overwhelmingly positive about the internet, using it for communicating with friends, for pleasure and fun and for research, whether for homework or a hobby' (2008: 118).

Have you ever played: Temple Run, Clash of Clans, Dragon Vale or Minecraft or any Wii or Xbox games? Your young client probably has and will most likely be able to beat your scores with ease.

Learning a new language

Do you know what a 'selfie' is or 'sexting'? Allow young clients to be the 'expert' by asking for a translation if they use an unfamiliar term. Childline also gives clear and easily available guides to these terms (www.childline.org.uk). For example: 'Sexting is when someone sends or receives a sexually explicit text, image or video on their mobile phone, usually in a text message'. The Childline information explains why a young person might get involved in sexting: reasons include being 'made to feel guilty' and being 'in love'. It goes on to ask young people to think, before they send the photo, what might happen to it, and gives suggestions of how to stop sexting and stay safe.

Be ready to enter into your client's world view; don't automatically judge 'screen time' or consider it as necessarily a problem. Recognise that young clients may be facing issues such as online bullying or they may be viewing inappropriate material.

Byron identified a 'generational digital divide'. As counsellors, we recognise that children may be in deeper water than they realise when in virtual worlds. Byron extends this analogy, saying that rather than being risk averse, not allowing children to get into 'deep water' online, we need to teach them to swim. To do this, we need to know about digital/virtual worlds. As counsellors, we need to recognise the risks and problems associated with new technologies without preaching or taking a critical parent position. If you feel out of your depth in the digital world, go online and just explore and play for a while. Ask a young person to show you the latest apps!

Consider how to respond when:

- young clients use online 'chat rooms', presuming those they meet online are exactly who they say they are
- there is online 'grooming'
- children and young people access unsuitable sites, including those that are violent or pornographic
- contact with others is confined to the 'virtual' world
- cyber bullying and exclusion are impacting on the client
- late nights online lead to a lack of sleep and an inability to concentrate.

Such problems are common when counselling children and young people and may lead to ethical dilemmas for the counsellor. For instance, online bullying and grooming are crimes. Counsellors need to understand and take seriously issues associated with young clients online. Regulation and parental controls are still absent for most children and young people in virtual worlds. Young clients need a safe place to share the 'deep water' they may have found themselves in. It is also necessary to remember that if a child or young person has been 'groomed' online, even if they have remained safe and discontinued the contact, there is a child protection issue.

Byron asks that we remember it is the particular circumstances of a child that puts them at risk online, rather than the internet itself being risky.

The counsellor's lack of knowledge of the 'generational digital divide' can be reduced through:

- familiarity with current research and thinking about online issues
- an openness to learn from the client
- being interested in new technologies
- challenging and supporting young people who may be out of their depth in virtual worlds.

CHAPTER SUMMARY

In this chapter, ethical dilemmas that often arise when counselling children and young people have been explored. A set of 'tools' enable the counsellor to approach dilemmas skilfully:

- Gain familiarity with the moral principles of the BACP Ethical Framework.
- Understand how ethical principles apply to specific issues that affect children and young people.
- Become adept at applying 'competing principles' to children and young people's issues for the best possible ethical outcome.
- Recognise that there are no easy answers to dilemmas and often no 'right' answer to be found.
- Understand child protection and safeguarding – sometimes the child or young person in the counselling room is not currently at risk, but their disclosure reveals risk to other children in that situation.
- Take into account the need for confidentiality and respect the privacy of counselling wherever possible.
- Remember that, at present, there is no mandatory duty to disclose and avoid automatic reporting if that is in the best interests of the young client and the context of counselling allows for a professional, ethical and considered judgement.

- Recognise that a dilemma may arise when the young client wants the counsellor to disclose and act on their behalf.

- Consider both school counsellors' independence and their need to be part of a team of professionals.

- Become familiar with the pleasures and pitfalls of young clients' life in virtual worlds. Recognise when it is necessary to take action to protect them.

REFERENCES

All Wales Child Protection Procedures (2008) Available at: awcpp.co.uk

British Association for Counselling and Psychotherapy (BACP) (2013) *Ethical Framework for Good Practice in Counselling and Psychotherapy*. Lutterworth: BACP.

Byron, T. (2008) Safer Children in a Digital World. Available at: www.gov.uk/dfe/byronreview

Clarke, P. (2004) *Clywch: Report of the Examination of the Children's Commissioner for Wales into Allegations of Child Sexual Abuse in a School Setting*. Swansea: Children's Commissioner for Wales.

Daniels, D. and Jenkins, P. (2010) *Therapy with Children: Children's Rights, Confidentiality and the Law*. London: Sage.

Department of Health (DoH) (1991) *The Children's Act 1989*. London: HMSO.

Gabriel, L. and Casemore, R. (2010) *P4 – Guidance for Ethical Decision Making: A Suggested Model*. Lutterworth: BACP.

Jenkins, P. (2013) 'Pelka's Law: reporting abuse', *Therapy Today*, 24(10): 33–5.

Johns, H. (2012) *Personal Development in Counsellor Training*, 2nd edn. London: Sage.

Joyce, P. and Sills, C. (2014) *Skills in Gestalt Counselling and Psychotherapy*, 3rd edn. London: Sage.

Martin, L. (2013) 'Self-harm: the solution, not the problem', *BACP Children and Young People*, June: 25–8.

McGinnis, S. with Jenkins, P. (2006) *Good Practice Guidelines for Counselling in Schools*, 4th edn. Lutterworth: BACP.

Owens, P., Springwood, B. and Wilson, M. (2012) *Creative Ethical Practice in Counselling and Psychotherapy*. London: Sage.

UNICEF (1989) *UN Convention on the Rights of the Child*. London: Children's Rights Development Unit.

Welsh Government (2008) *All Wales Child Protection Procedures*. Cardiff: Welsh Government.

Withnall, A. (2013) 'Health expert calls for age of consent to be lowered to 15', *Independent*, 17 November. Available at: www.independent.co.uk/news/uk/home-news/health-expert-calls-for-age-of-consent-to-be-lowered-to-15-8945235.html

LEGAL CASE

Gillick *v.* West Norfolk AHA (1985) 3 All ER 402 (1986) AC1127.

7

SKILFUL PLAY FOR COUNSELLORS

INTRODUCTION

This chapter offers ideas and information for the counsellor who wants to include play and ways of communicating that don't just involve sitting and talking. The chapter is not about play therapy but does seek to show the therapeutic value of play.

Counsellors often find they are working in multi-functional rooms, not in well-equipped playrooms. If they have play equipment, it is often portable – a basket, a box or items from the boot of the car.

When reading, researching or receiving training on how to play with children and young people in counselling, a feeling of frustration can arise from a lack of play space, equipment or resources. Play materials do not need to cost much or come from specialist suppliers. Simple items such as blank paper and crayons, small pots of children's modelling clay from the local supermarket, a pack of cards or imagination games that require no materials at all can be part of skilful play in counselling.

Relevant methods of play and how theories of play, both directed and non-directed, can be put skilfully into practice without a dedicated playroom, are the subject of this chapter.

Included are:

- a guide to counsellors gaining confidence and ability with play in counselling

- exploring the counsellor's inner free child

- consideration of how different modalities might approach play in counselling

- how to choose and integrate ways of playing

- what we may learn about young clients from observing how they play

- a counsellor's home grown play 'kit' – and what it includes

- using emotional literacy games to explore feelings

- positives and pitfalls of play; how to start and when to stop; winning and losing; taking turns

- taking made items home and displays in the counselling room; preserving confidentiality with play
- skills in playing with younger children and with adolescents
- using clay, art materials and toy animals/dolls
- playing card games, board games and jigsaws for digression and enjoyment.

GAINING CONFIDENCE AND ABILITY WITH PLAY

Many counsellors have had little experience with play in the context of counselling when they begin counselling children and young people. Counselling is primarily a 'talking' therapy and yet we will have young clients who are unable or unwilling to talk. Adult clients have usually chosen to come to counselling and expect to come and tell their story. Children and young people are far more mixed in their pre-knowledge of the counselling process. Ask them how they are and the answer may be 'fine' or a shrug of the shoulders and a blank look at you. At first, their counsellor seems similar to other adults who are trying to get them to 'behave', 'be quiet' or 'do their homework'.

The use of play in counselling can bridge the gap – the wide space between 'adult counsellor' and 'child or adolescent client'. There is a sense of equality in the process of playing together. Clients may feel on safer 'ground', recognising the 'rules' or the 'shape' of the play, whereas talking about their personal life is likely to be very unfamiliar to most young clients.

If the counsellor is unfamiliar with play as a therapeutic process, there can be some reticence to begin playing within counselling. Young clients will 'pick up' feelings of uncertainty in their counsellor and will be less likely to engage with the play materials. Counsellors can initially question the value of play and hold concerns about whether the 'tasks' of counselling are being fulfilled if we are using soft clay, miniature animals, playing cards or board games with our young clients rather than talking about their problems.

Later in the chapter, we will consider methods of play, what counsellors can learn and how to find the appropriate level of play for different clients. In this section, we will consider how counsellors can become more confident with play. Let's begin by considering your relationship with play.

MINDFUL MOMENT

Take a moment, close your eyes and bring to mind a time when you were playing as a child. Who was there? Were you playing alone or with others? How old were you? What were you feeling?

THE PLAY JOURNAL

REFLECTIVE ACTIVITY: PREPARATION FOR PLAY — THE PLAY JOURNAL

- Obtain a blank journal or sheets of paper without lines on the page.

- Start to write down or draw/paint pictures in your journal of your own experiences of playing.

- Example: My first memory was 'American skipping' with elastic round our ankles in the school playground. A second memory was of being at home in the dining room with china animals being made into a choir; in this memory I was playing alone.

- There are few 'rules' with this activity, but it is useful if you can remember your childhood play. If you can't access a memory of childhood play, then write how you feel about not remembering and any reasons why you might not be able to recall this aspect of your past.

- Note any sounds, songs or music that you remember from 'play time'. I immediately hear the theme of *Andy Pandy*, a children's TV show that I watched during my early childhood.

- Memories may 'flood in' or be hard to access; note down anything you can remember.

- Now begin to note any feelings that accompany the memories. If this activity stimulates strong feelings, do get support with this.

- If possible, share strong feelings or memories with a supervisor/trusted colleague/partner or in your own counselling or therapy.

- Note whether play feels like a distant memory or if you still enjoy play and have fun in your life.

- Return to this journal when you have experiences with play when counselling. Preserve the anonymity of young clients, but note your experiences and choices. The journal will become a resource that you can develop and return to.

Keeping a play journal will enable:

- empathic responses: once you have clarified your own relationship with play, you can be 'in the shoes' of your client more easily when playing with them

- self-awareness: when emotions arise during play in the counselling room, we can recognise them, whether they are our emotions or our client's or a mixture of both.

I remember when I first visited my daughter's 'kindergarten' in a Rudolph Steiner school in Wales. The kindergarten is a beautiful circular building with a grass roof deep in a quiet valley. It has nooks and crannies, simple toys and dressing-up clothes, all in soft colours. It is a child-centred environment designed for the young child to gently transition between the world of home and that of school. Having never been to anything remotely like this in my own childhood, I felt a sense of loss sweep over me. My 'inner child' wanted to stay and be nurtured there.

Awareness of relationship with play

Shining the light of self-awareness on experiences like these, noting them in the play journal, understanding and coming to terms with both enjoyment and loss in childhood play is a vital step for counsellors before beginning play with young clients. Perhaps we had to 'fight' for toys with siblings or were chastised for being 'messy' or 'dirty' as children. We may have joyful memories of freedom too. Bringing all this into awareness will make us much more skilful with young clients. It's easy to be 'caught unaware' if our childhood play experiences remain unexamined.

Awareness of difference

Our client may have a very different understanding of play to ours. If we haven't considered this, then we could unintentionally misjudge them. An example of this is a counsellor wanting their client to go out and play more because they had such a good time playing outside as a child. The client's circumstances may be so different that going out to play is inappropriate in their case. It may be frightening, upsetting or even dangerous for a young client to be encouraged to play in this way. The counsellor's inappropriate encouragement to 'go outside and have fun' will be confusing and potentially upsetting for a young client who is, for example, being bullied in the playground.

Purpose of a play journal
- Reflect on your practice of play in counselling.
- Share play experiences and ideas from your journal with other counsellors.
- Note down ideas and methods to use with clients.
- Recognise strengths and areas where more learning and practice are needed with play, both in your own life and in counselling.
- Develop your inner 'free child'.

Activity: Developing your inner 'free child'

The following are examples of how you can find a childlike quality often lost or suppressed by adults:

- Be spontaneous.
- Tell jokes.
- Eat something you really like, rather than something you 'should' eat.
- Take some small risks, e.g. buy a new piece of clothing that you like but wouldn't normally wear.
- Get something wrong and see the funny side.
- Dance, sing or paint a picture.
- Sleep for as long as you want to.
- If you feel cross, grumpy, excited or happy, enter into that feeling with as much energy as you can.
- Say 'no' to something you ought to do but don't want to.
- Ignore this list of activities because you are not interested in doing them!

Knowing ourselves in play

Once we have more knowledge about ourselves in the process of play within counselling, then our confidence will begin to develop. The emphasis is on being playful and spontaneous, which is similar to congruence – being with and acting on your feelings without modification.

We recognise as adults that modification and adaptation must take place in order to live harmoniously with others. We cannot always have what we want. As adults, we have often lost touch with what it is that we want. Children and young people have much more of a sense of their own needs and what they want, but we teach them to adapt these needs to fit in with family and school life. In counselling, play can allow deep needs to be expressed. Some needs are simple. Young clients may need to:

- smile and relax
- feel cared for and noticed
- be able to express angry, sad and joyful feelings
- dream, rest or be silent

- be listened to
- receive attention and understanding for being themselves.

These aims for play in counselling can offer solace to a troubled or misunderstood child or young person.

NON-DIRECTED OR DIRECTED PLAY

Play in counselling can either be directed, non-directed or a mixture of both. The style that you choose may be based on your modality (see Chapter 4) or on what you consider a particular client needs.

One way to know what is the best play activity for your client is to allow them to make the choice of what they play with. There are materials that are easy to obtain and children and young people can choose from what is made available to them in counselling.

Choice

Letting a child or young person choose their game or toy is a helpful way of building the relationship and participation in counselling. The game or toy can become a conduit, a method of communication which may enable them to reveal what is troubling and difficult in their lives.

DIFFERENT MODALITIES' APPROACH TO PLAY

- A psychodynamic counsellor's perspective on play is likely to be based on early attachment and the symbolic nature of play. It is important in this approach not to interpret the choices made in play. 'Play, above all, is the space where learning takes place at the child's pace, with the child's agenda' (Hopper 2007: 66).
- Person-centred counsellors may wish to only use non-directed play based on the belief that what the child or young person brings to the play will allow them to experience growth when the right conditions are met (Axline 1989).
- Solution-focused, goal-oriented, cognitive-behavioural counsellors are likely to find directed play more suitable.
- Narrative counsellors may focus on 'thickening' – new ways of understanding the young client's story through play.
- Integrative counsellors may be able to draw on many styles of play in counselling. Geldard and Geldard (2008) offer a model of counselling children that includes five phases drawn from five different modalities:
  o Phase 1: Client-centred therapy – the child joins with the counsellor.
  o Phase 2: Gestalt therapy – the client works on awareness, releasing emotions and dealing with resistance.

- Phase 3: Narrative therapy – the client develops a different view of themselves.
- Phase 4: Cognitive-behavioural therapy – the child challenges unhelpful thoughts and looks at options.
- Phase 5: Behaviour therapy: the client experiences new behaviours and their consequences.

Using Geldard and Geldard's (2008) model in play offers a method that uses directed play whilst integrating client-centred aspects.

Directed play

There are fully directed ways of playing in counselling where the counsellor makes the 'rules' and the child joins in. There can be fun and good therapeutic outcomes from this type of play. It can be a rewarding and enjoyable experience for the young client. An advantage of this style of play would be the child's familiarity with it from their classroom and home life where rules and guidance are usually given.

Non-directed play

In non-directed approaches to play, the child is free to choose from any play materials available. The manner in which they interact with the play materials can give the counsellor a great deal of information about the client's 'inner world'. The counsellor may want to join in, if invited to do so, or just notice and reflect on the choices made by the child or young person.

It is helpful for the counsellor to understand where they are on a continuum between using directed and non-directed methods of play in counselling, rather than just choosing a game and playing it.

MINDFUL MOMENT: PLAY WITH MINIATURE ANIMALS — BEGINNERS' MIND

Before reading the exercise below, take a moment to stop and breathe.

Put three miniature animals on a table in front of you. See them as if for the first time. Pick them up, smell them, feel their shape. Close your eyes and hold them in your hands. Open your eyes and place the little animals back on the table. Move them around.

What do you notice? Are you enjoying this moment? Do you like one animal better than another? Do you like how they smell and feel or not?

Note your responses without judging them. It's your experience that matters.

> # CASE EXAMPLE: SANDRA PLAYS WITH MINIATURE ANIMALS
>
> Sandra is 8 years old, she has been bullied at two schools she has attended and now her parents are considering moving her to a third school. Her teachers are concerned that moving her again will be making her situation worse not better. Sandra was adopted at the age of 3 by her current family; the exact circumstances of her years with her birth family are not clear. Sandra moves between being shy and withdrawn into sudden outbursts of deep crying, shouting and hitting out when provoked. Her teachers find her willing to learn, but she seems to have great difficulty in making friends, preferring to play alone.
>
> ### Information from Sandra's teachers
>
> According to her teachers, the other children find her 'odd' and her parents are 'over-protective', wanting to undo the problems that are clearly from her early home life by giving her a calm and forgiving home environment now. Whilst this works well for Sandra when she is the only child present, it has not helped her integrate with other children. The teachers do not think she is the victim of a campaign of bullying; rather they have noticed that when other children are trying to get Sandra to join in their games, she refuses and moves away. Recently though, they have had to intervene when a small group of girls were calling Sandra names and telling her to go away when she stood near them. One was holding her nose and calling Sandra 'smelly'. Sandra then hit the girl who called her 'smelly'. The parents of this girl complained about Sandra's behaviour to the school. Everyone is concerned to make sure that this does not happen again and the teachers are keeping a close watch on the situation.
>
> ### Sandra's second session
>
> Sandra comes for her second session of counselling and is interacting well with you. You need to get more understanding of how she is in groups and, as she has expressed a love for animals, you make sure the miniature animals are readily available in the counselling room.
>
> The animals could represent relationships in Sandra's life, so do you suggest this to her or not? The choice is between directing her play with the miniature animals and allowing her to freely play with them as she chooses.

Below are different ways for Sandra to interact with the miniature animals based on a variety of approaches to play in counselling.

1 An integrative approach to playing with the animals

Geldard and Geldard (2008) give an example of how you could direct Sandra's play. They suggest you explain to your young client that you are going to play with the animals in a special way:

'First of all, I would like you to choose an animal that is most like you.'

When the animal is chosen, questions are asked to gain information about what the young client thinks is the personality of that animal – a monkey is cheeky or agile, a horse calm and strong, for example. This exercise may be extended by asking Sandra to choose animals to represent family members or her classmates in order to gain insight as to how she sees herself in these groups.

A great deal of information can be gained in this way, asking the child or young person to move animals into various positions and noticing responses, anxieties or pleasure in different constellations of the animals. Always refer to the animals by their names – 'the horse' or 'the monkey' – not by the name of the person they are representing.

Skills for an integrative, directed style of play include the following:

- Tell the child/young person they are to choose a miniature animal to represent themselves and to represent each of the others they are in relationship with.
- Ask your young client to tell you about the personality of each miniature animal.
- Give instructions on how to move the miniature animals, e.g. closer together or further apart.
- Notice reluctance, anxiety or pleasure in these changes.
- Ask open questions and reflect on what you notice.

2 A psychodynamic approach to playing with the animals

In this non-directed approach, to discover more about Sandra she would be allowed to play with the miniature animals as she wished. There would be an acceptance of whatever she chose in the play alongside observation of her playing.

Hopper explains that: 'Play needs to come from the child's inner self and not be shaped to conform to external constraints' (2007: 65). She goes on to say that although a child may not resent it if others control and direct the play, that child is likely to conform to the agenda of the counsellor, trying to find the 'right' answer rather than their own 'internal locus' of control. Play needs to 'have the quality of drawing from the child the precious parts of himself that lie within' (2007: 66).

Self-directed play

If Sandra plays in this way, she might choose, for example, to hide some animals, cover them with clothes, sing to them, put them to sleep, give them food or endless varieties of activities that may not make immediate sense to the counsellor but *do* make sense to Sandra.

What is the counsellor's role in this play?

Mindful observation The counsellor will notice and observe the play, allowing it to change and develop over time. The young client may want the counsellor to take a role in the play; if this is the case, the client must always be allowed to take the lead. So much will be communicated to the counsellor in observing the play in this way and the young client will realise the deep level of acceptance, that there is no way to 'get it wrong'. There may simply need to be some limits based on the environment of the counselling room. Throwing the animals around may be unacceptable in rooms where there are glass panels, for example. Counsellors need to be realistic as to what is possible in the space where they are playing. It is possible though to allow the principles of 'self-directed play' to take place in counselling. The results can be deeply moving when there is a creative allowing of whatever needs to be expressed.

The tiger knocks the deer down Sandra may, for example, play with a large tiger that knocks over a small deer again and again. She says 'naughty' every time she pushes the tiger into the deer. She sternly tells the deer to 'stand up straight' each time she knocks it over, she handles the deer roughly and is very angry with it. She tells the small deer to 'behave' and 'stop crying or I will give you something to cry for'. At times, she glances at you quizzically, then returns to the 'game', the tiger getting more and more violent towards the deer. Whilst it may be tempting to comment on this or try and protect the deer in some way, it is necessary to remember that this may be the only opportunity Sandra has to reveal her innermost hurt.

As counsellors observing, we don't know if the deer represents Sandra or someone else in her early experience. We don't know if this actually happened or if it is imaginary or partly both. What we do know is that Sandra is choosing to play in this way.

Near the end of the session, Sandra begins to comfort the little deer and tells it that it is really the tiger who is bad. Once again, as counsellors, we need to allow this to take place, recognising our own feelings of sadness or relief that the deer is now being comforted.

Play requires time This way of being with play does require time, so we may recognise that the limits of our circumstances do not allow for this type of exploration.

Skills in self-directed play from a psychodynamic perspective include:

- allowing play to come from the child or young person's 'inner self'
- observation without intervention, holding 'a completely clear space for the child' (Hooper 2007: 67)
- giving time to allow the development of play and changes to take place.

3 A Gestalt approach to playing with the animals

In a Gestalt approach to play, there would be encouragement to 'be' the miniature animals in the 'here and now' or express what was missing in a scene with miniature animals. There is a difference between asking what the miniature animal is 'like', as described earlier in a more integrative and directed form of play, and the Gestalt approach of 'being' the animal and speaking in the present tense, as in this example, as an angry tiger or a 'frightened' deer.

Sandra speaks as the tiger If Sandra can speak as the angry, violent tiger, it could help her to release feelings that would be hard to accept in other circumstances. When 'being' the tiger, Sandra might say: 'I am angry and I am very strong. I can hurt you and there is nothing you can do about it.' This is an expression of the way she was treated in her early life. Sandra's teachers have seen her act aggressively when she was threatened. It is a common occurrence for children and young people who have been treated in violent or aggressive ways to then act this out on others. The result of this is that the victim turns into a persecutor and may find that they are punished or excluded for their behaviour.

There is a tragic element in the life of a child who has been the victim of abuse and who then 'acts' out in unacceptable ways that put them in the wrong. The Gestalt method of being the 'bad' tiger for a moment gives an outlet for these 'internalised' feelings of badness or aggression.

Skills in Gestalt-based play in counselling include:

◆ noticing and being present

◆ speaking in the 'here and now', e.g. being the miniature animal

◆ considering what or who is missing in play (Mortola 2006).

4 A client-centred approach to playing with the animals

In Chapter 4, the eight principles of play therapy (Axline 1989) were included in the section on person-centred counselling. These principles can be applied to the case of Sandra and her play with miniature animals. We have established in this case study that Sandra wants to play with the miniature animals. If she did not, then there would be no question within the client-centred way of playing that they would be introduced.

Not compromising values by 'forcing' Sandra to play Axline (1989) gives an example of this when she writes of how a counsellor or therapist can compromise their client-centred values, even when simply attempting to establish rapport, by forcing, cajoling, complimenting and wheedling in order to get the young client to play. Here, we identify the differences between an integrative counsellor who has person-centred values and the counsellor who is fully client centred. The client-centred counsellor allows the child or young person to go at their own pace, accepts them completely and trusts that within this environment of the counselling room, the young client then begins to respect the therapy as they are respected within it.

In the case of Sandra and her play with the miniature animals, this fully client-centred approach would mean offering her that deep respect that shows we have a belief that she will begin to resolve her own problems through the play. It is important to remember that there are limitations to the freedom that can be allowed when playing in the counselling room. Young clients are not allowed to threaten or attack their counsellor or continually break equipment. If Sandra did break something in play, particularly if she broke the leg off the tiger, for example, it would be important not to reject her or be angry whilst establishing that breaking play materials is not acceptable.

Responding to challenges Responses to these types of challenges whilst playing with a child or young person in counselling are usefully considered in advance, but most often it is the mindful response in the moment that will be required. Keeping calm and being comfortable with the inevitable uncertainty present when allowing a child or young person to play in a non-directed way are skills developed over time.

Skills in client-centred non-directed play include the following:

- Accept the child or young person as they are.
- Don't compromise a client-centred approach by complimenting or cajoling the child into participating in play.
- Remember that trust and mutual respect are key to this approach to play.
- Know your limitations and don't allow personal attacks or repeated destructive play that breaks the play materials.
- Enjoy the uncertainty and be alongside your young client in how they choose to play.

ADAPTING PLAY METHODS TO FIT THE CIRCUMSTANCES OF COUNSELLING

A counsellor's day in a primary school

Imagine you have just started counselling one day a week at your local primary school. This is your third week and you have seen five young clients, all aged 10 or 11. Your remit is to focus on the transition between primary and secondary school. You are an integrative counsellor with lots of experience as both a play leader and a youth worker.

A suitable room?

You are offered the deputy head's office as your counselling room for the day. You are aware that the deputy head has made a big concession in offering her room and you don't want to comment about the drawbacks of using this room for counselling. You have been told that there are no other rooms available and you want to get on with the job. In the room are lots of worksheets piled up, keys hanging on hooks on the wall and lists of children's names on notice boards. You begin by carefully moving everything on to the highest shelves available, remembering where everything has come from to replace it at the end of the day.

Your integrative approach means holding client-centred values whilst feeling comfortable with elements of directed play in counselling. You are aware too that different methods may suit each of your clients.

Mike

One young client, Mike, is a very active boy and he likes to throw a soft ball as hard as he can at the wall. You feel that this is a very useful activity for him. You know his home life holds lots of frustrations for him and it is palpable that Mike is expressing these when throwing the ball at the wall over and over again. You are, however, anxious that items belonging to the deputy head will be moved or accidently broken. You don't know whether to intervene and direct his play or allow him the free expression that is clearly his self-directed choice. You settle on allowing the play to continue, but your self-awareness tells you that your own anxiety is affecting the way play progresses. You think Mike knows you are anxious and will therefore 'test' you by throwing the ball just next to items belonging to the deputy head.

Molly

Later in the day, Molly arrives for counselling. Molly lives in the local women's refuge with her mum and younger sister. Molly describes her mum as both 'cross' and 'strict'. Molly is afraid of getting dirty at school because her mum will be very angry. She wants to play with the play clay. You have kept the play clay in its separate colours, the colours are bright and inviting and most young clients enjoy choosing the colours and putting them back in their own pots. Molly, however, wants to mix them all up into a brown colour. You feel this is therapeutic for her and her one and only place where she is allowed to be 'messy' for a while. You are, however, disappointed as your clay is changed into a brown lump, never to return to the bright colours you started with. You think about the children coming later in the day and wonder if they are being disadvantaged by allowing Molly this freedom to mix the colours.

Andrea

Andrea is your last client of the day; she is in foster care and the complex circumstances of her life mean that she will probably be unable to return home in the foreseeable future to either her mother, who is considered unsuitable by social services, or her step-father, who loves her and wants to adopt her. Andrea's mother has made accusations of abuse against her step-father and although Andrea doesn't corroborate these and wants to live with her step-father, the decision has been taken that this is not to be allowed at present. Andrea has been in five foster placements in the last six months. You see her at the end of the day because she has great difficulty in leaving the counselling room. The head has told you that you are the first person Andrea has engaged with, she refuses to talk to social workers and in class is withdrawn, though above average in academic ability. When allowing Andrea to choose how to play in counselling, she takes the deputy head's keys off their hook on the wall and hides them at the bottom of the play box. At each stage of this activity, she stops and stares at you, noting your reactions at every moment. You are torn between wanting to allow her to continue and recognising that these keys are not yours and must not be lost or damaged. You make a mental note to remove them before next week, but right now you don't want to stop Andrea's play. You find the hiding of keys to be a poignant expression of her difficult circumstances where her life is so out of control and she has no 'key' to resolving it. You wonder if she has been locked in rooms as she wants to 'pretend' to lock you in one part of the room whilst she is in another.

Two more clients that day

Your other two clients that day have chosen drawing and just talking with you, both highly suitable activities for the environment of this particular counselling room. Mike, Molly and Andrea have all made you question whether you need to direct them in their play more because of the room you are counselling in, rather than because this would be best for them in their expression through play.

Whilst you are managing and learning through your experience of play with clients in this way, there are skilful practices that can prevent some of the anxieties and risks evident in the day outlined above:

- As a counsellor with children and young people, have basic requirements for where you offer play in counselling. These need to be explained to the school or agency where you will be counselling.

- You and your young client need a quiet and safe space to play.

- Be clear, assertive and yet adaptable about what is needed.

- Be prepared to say 'no' to counselling in an entirely unsuitable space. Ask for adaptations to be made if necessary. In the above case, perhaps more preparation of the room would have helped – a box for personal and private objects to be placed in for the day, for example.

- Stay within the limitations of not allowing violent or destructive play.

- Know that you are able to stop the play if necessary, if, for example, a safety issue arises.

- Choose a more directed style of play if you find you are anxious with non-directed play or you have very short time limits on the counselling you can offer.

- Remember that counselling is primarily about the relationship between client and counsellor. This applies in play as much as in any other activity, so choose methods that will not inhibit your ability to be present with your young client.

- If you do have a safe and comfortable room to play in with young clients in counselling, then decide on the methods of play and play materials you want to use, relax and enjoy the process.

- Recognise that the nature of play is that it is not entirely predictable in its outcomes. The therapeutic value lies in allowing the young client to have some choices even if the play is directed.

- Remember that holding client-centred values means keeping young clients like Mike, Molly and Andrea safe when they are playing. Hurting themselves or breaking something in counselling would be counter-therapeutic. We may need to limit the play we offer in order to fit with the counselling environment.

- Choose how you are going to offer play in counselling, practise methods with colleagues or in other settings and then introduce them into counselling.

CHOOSING PLAY MATERIALS

What does a counsellor need to play with young clients in counselling? The first answer to this question is: Nothing at all.

Play requiring no equipment

Emotional literacy images

How does it look and feel to be happy, sad, angry, jealous, depressed or excited? Some children do not have a good grasp on the language of feelings so playing and experimenting with what emotions look like, sound like and feel like can be useful at times. Sometimes a child will be very familiar with sadness but never express anger. Learning safe ways to express being angry without hitting out or hurting anyone can be a very helpful skill for young clients to learn.

A reason to play could be that you have recognised whilst counselling a young client that they don't express emotion easily. Start with a guessing game:

Say: I'm going to show you a feeling and I want you to guess what it is.

Make a sad face, let your body slump in the chair and make a 'sad' sound like a sigh or groan. Hold the position for a moment and ask your client what they see. Give prompts like:

- What do you see on my face?

- What do you see my body is like?

- What are the sounds I am making?

Repeat the position and help with responses if they are not very forthcoming.

Ask your client to show you sadness. Their interpretation will probably be different to yours. Make it clear that it doesn't have to be the same as yours or it is possible they will just copy you.

Next you both show your version of an emotion to each other at the same time. Freeze the postures and move your eyes only to look at the other person's 'image' of that emotion. Notice what is happening in your own body and face as well as that of your client. Let go of the posture, shake out to make sure you don't get stuck in that emotion and then talk for a while about what it was like to express emotions in that way. Different cultures will express emotions in a variety of ways. Make it clear that differences are to be encouraged. The purpose of this game is to become familiar with a 'language' of emotions. Later in the counselling, if a young client is having difficulty in expressing how they feel, you can just say, 'Would you like to show me the image rather than speak about this?' This game is also fun and informative in groups (Dowsett 2009).

Expressing strong emotions Be aware that expressing strong emotions such as anger or grief in this way can bring them to the surface quickly. Note too that if you show an angry face to a young client this could be scary for them. Don't start with anger unless you find this is specifically what is needed. The one time you might begin with anger is if your client is an adolescent who is experiencing anger or aggression problems but never shows this aspect of themselves in counselling.

Imaginary superhero/heroine Create an imaginary character with your young client who is able to intervene to help them when they have a difficult memory. This game is useful if a child has nightmares based on a situation that they have now been removed from but which is very real and present, either when they are asleep or in waking 'flashbacks'. This game could be extended into drawing but it can be left at imagination.

It is *very* important not to encourage a child to relive a past trauma if they don't want to do so or you have not been specifically trained to work with them in that way. It is equally important not to deny the presence of intrusive thoughts and feelings from past trauma or to try and 'gloss' over them.

Introduce the idea tentatively – the way you do this will depend on the age of your client. Give the idea: 'What if you put someone into your memory/dream/flashback who can help you get safe? This isn't a real person, they are magic, invincible and completely on your side. They might be able to cast invisibility spells, to give you wings or be so strong that any bad person is stopped from hurting you.'

This game might also lead to the creation of a new story for the young client with a happier ending than the one they actually experienced. Never denying or belittling what happened in the past, this activity can create a resource for living in the present without the pain of the past constantly invading their thoughts and feelings.

Identify what their superhero or heroine looks like, sounds like, what they say and do. Allow your client to create the character as far as possible, though you might add a few qualities, in the style of a fairy godmother/father as wishes for them. The young often have a great imagination and this can be utilised to help them in recovery from very difficult events.

When they have created their super-heroine/hero, ask them to bring up a memory of something mildly unpleasant, such as a lesson they don't like or a check-up at the dentist. Firmly discourage going straight into abuse or other very upsetting memories. This is a first practice. Find out if they can imagine their super-heroine/hero alongside them in the mildly unpleasant memory. Check out how the character they have invented helps them. You need to observe your young client carefully and ascertain if they are finding this helpful. It might be amusing, and they may feel protected and more able to function in adverse circumstances.

In a later session, ask if they have thought of their superhero/heroine, see if they report feeling helped when they were feeling low, and then use the technique with more difficult memories. Make sure your client understands that an imaginary character cannot protect them in 'real-life' danger. This way of working is helpful for flashbacks and intrusive memories of past events.

Relaxation and breathing Children and young people can be very tense and stressed and activities that just slow everything down can be helpful. A moment of quietness at the beginning of a session after a child has raced into the room, counting three to breathe in and three to breathe out, is a good activity *if* it is made fun and enjoyable rather than something a client is asked to do in order to 'make' them calm down.

Young people who are tired and have exam stress can value being taken through a 'body scan' where each part of the body is relaxed in turn. It is advisable for counsellors to have had plenty of experience with this type of activity themselves before using it with young clients. Whilst relaxation can seem straightforward, it may have unexpected outcomes such as frightening thoughts or feelings arising whilst relaxing. In general, this is an activity to be avoided with traumatised clients and those with mental health disorders (Adler-Tapia 2012). Used appropriately, relaxation activities can be very enjoyable and helpful for those simply feeling wound up or exhausted from their everyday lives.

Play and creative activities

Board games/jigsaws and playing cards Most counsellors will be familiar with how to play some board and card games. These, as with jigsaws, are very useful for taking turns and require a basic level of listening to each other. Such activities can be used as a way of communicating and establishing relationships. Often, talking will flow much more if a game like this is taking place. Geldard, Geldard and Yin Foo (2013: 251) suggest that games allow the child 'to experience, experiment with and practice responses to tasks involving communication, social interaction and the solving of problems'. Whilst we may not be actively looking for these outcomes in our counselling, it is useful to recognise them as possibilities. If the focus of our counselling is more person-centred, we may want to join in with our client, experience winning and losing and through this deepen our connection with them.

One counsellor in a school introduced a young person to a new card game that became the latest 'fashion' in that whole school year! We need to be aware of the responsibility that we have in our choice of games that we introduce.

Poetry, lyrics, stories and creative writing Poetry and song lyrics are a good medium to connect with the 'inner condition' of troubled children and young people. The question 'is there a song in your mind right now?' can reveal how a young client is feeling and help to alleviate feelings of shame or embarrassment about expressing emotions. Asking young clients to write down random words about how they feel during the week and bring these to counselling can be approached playfully and creatively. Activities like this work best when they are optional and not 'homework'.

Therapeutic story writing, transposing real-life characters into creatures or fairytale characters is an excellent medium for some young clients to express themselves (Bolton et al. 2004). (See the counsellor's play kit for examples from practice later in this chapter.)

The Freedom Writer's Diary (Grunwell 2009) is suitable for older teenagers and shows the power of truthful journal writing to create change for young people. Maya Angelou (2010) writes of her own journey with poetry after becoming mute due to childhood trauma. During the silence, 'poems would play through her mind like invisible friends' (Rosen 2009: 22).

Drawing and painting There are many activities that are suitable as play in counselling that involve drawing and painting. Doodling and 'free' drawing can be very useful with older children and young people. You can ask your young client to say anything they like about what they have drawn. At the other end of the spectrum, there are more structured activities, some of which are described in Chapter 4, such as drawing lifelines and pictures of family members.

Drawings and paintings can be carefully stored and shown to a supervisor to help in understanding that particular client or as a record of progress. Some young clients don't have anywhere safe to keep pictures at home, so the counsellor creating a record through the counselling with their young client can be a great resource.

Preserving anonymity with play materials Take care to preserve anonymity if pictures and results of other creative activities are displayed in the counselling room. Whilst it would be my personal preference not to display in this way, because children might copy what they see rather than have ideas come from their own experience, I understand that some counsellors find displays valuable in offering examples and allowing all their clients to feel included, creating a sense of belonging in the counselling room.

There is a great deal of information available about play therapy with children and young people (McMahon 2005). Use resources wisely and remember that young clients are not to be experimented on. Careful thought and practice are needed before play is used for the first time in counselling.

Activities that require more specific equipment such as sand trays have not been included in this chapter. They will, however, be appropriately used by some counsellors with children and young people who have been trained in play therapy techniques and have access to suitable facilities (Carey 2008).

A COUNSELLOR'S PLAY KIT

In the following, two counsellors who are experienced with play with children and young people in counselling give an explanation of the materials they use, how to use them and which clients they are suitable for. The examples show how the simplest of 'tools', like a photocopied 'snakes and ladders' board or an old magazine with pictures, can be utilised to create play that is inventive and very helpful to the young client.

The first counsellor offers an example of a play kit that is easy to carry around and shows how play is integrated into the counselling. She begins by naming the toy or game and then explains how it is used:

Slinky: this appeals to younger teens and children and brings some joy to them

Tangle: this is about fun and keeping young clients' hands busy, but is also useful for topics like being confused and 'all tangled up'

Play clay: this is fun, comforting, very useful for metaphor work and for connecting with the child within

Pick-up sticks: mostly unknown to a generation of children used to fancy electronic toys, this is a simple game of skill which few know but all seem to love. It is great to play when children and young people need to settle before going back to a lesson, or when they need to engage in a playful activity, not just talking. I don't use it in my 'special educational needs' (SEN) school as it requires dexterity but I use it with primary and secondary children. Rules can be simplified or made more complex. It is very useful to observe here how clients learn and handle rules/outcomes

Snakes and ladders: this is mostly played with younger children and young people with SEN. I use photocopies of the board so we can colour in the bits on which we land and take things slowly. Mainly we say something that makes us happy if we land on a ladder and unhappy if we land on a snake. My board has arrows and we can say anything/make a wish if we land on those

Salt and chalk jars: this involves a child choosing a coloured chalk, giving the colour a meaning, grinding it into a scoop of salt, pouring that into a jar and then starting again. The jar fills with a landscape of emotions/thoughts. It is not so easy to cart around, but is messy, creative, fabulous for facilitating communication, sorting out emotions, allowing positivity to be expressed, containing trauma and giving shape/colour to formless thoughts/feelings. Glitter and tea leaves are useful additions; wet wipes are a must.

This example shows how the counsellor's practice brings fluency with play. The choice of play materials used with different client groups is illuminating. This counsellor works in a variety of school settings throughout her week and takes care to pick a suitable activity for her clients.

The second counsellor shows how whole sessions can be dedicated to one play activity and how an activity might stretch over more than one session.

Use of play techniques in counselling

Identity parade

You will need:

- A3 or larger paper
- pictures cut out from magazines or printed off from the internet.

Method Spend time collecting pictures from magazines/the internet of celebrities who are currently in the public eye and may be relevant to the age group that you are working with. This can be done before the counselling begins to save time or can be done with the child in session to involve them in the process, which may also give you an opportunity to talk about the qualities of people and themselves.

Working with the child, line up the pictures horizontally in the middle of the paper as if they were in an identity parade, allowing space above and below the pictures to add anything else (do not glue them down as they may move as the session goes on). Ask the child to group the people together into different categories such as funny people, successful people, positive/negative role models, etc. These may change as discussions begin.

When people have been grouped, discuss individually what each of these people mean to the child when they look at them and ask if there is anyone in their lives who acts/looks like this. Ask the child: if they had to place themselves anywhere in the parade, where would it be and why?

My script

You will need:

- images of a wide range of films
- paper and pen.

Method Before the session, prepare sheets of pictures from magazines or the internet of different films in different genres relevant to the age of the child being worked with. If you don't want to do pictures, then you can just list the names of the films.

In the session, ask the child to look through the different genres and ask which ones they are mostly drawn to, discussing the reasons behind this.

Next, work with the child to try and create their own life in an imaginative film. If they had to portray their life for others to understand how they see the world, what would the setting be? Who would be in it? What would the beginning, middle and end be like? What would the audience take from the film afterwards?

If they had to remake the original film, what changes would they make? How would they do this? This part of rewriting the script can sometimes be enough to facilitate change.

The story of two halves

You will need:

- an exercise book/notebook
- pens and, if available, art equipment.

Method Ask the child if they want to write the following story in a book or print it from the computer and create the book digitally.

Begin exploring how they feel about their lives and what have been the good parts and the not so good parts of their lives up until now. For some children, this may be too threatening, especially if the child has been through very adverse circumstances. In situations like this, give the child the option to make up a character, rather than writing about themselves, and then write a description about this character. Next, ask for another character that is the opposite type of person (maybe the shadow side of the original character).

Split the book into two halves and ask the child to start writing basic facts about the two characters, or the good and not so good parts of their lives, in each section, and then to write about the past, present and future in each half of the book. Depending on the age of the child, it may be easier for the counsellor to write down what the child is saying.

After this has been completed, ask the child:

- to give it a title
- what sort of person this book would be good for
- what it was like writing it
- which of the two sides of the book was easier to write and which was most difficult
- if they were to write another book/other books what this/these would be called.

These play activities are creative and will offer lots of opportunity for learning and reflection. They also allow the child or young person to make choices and decisions within the play. This experienced counsellor is noting, too, when these play activities would not be suitable.

Landreth (2012: 9) offers the insight: 'For children to "play out" their experiences and feelings is the most natural dynamic and self-healing process in which they can engage'. As counsellors, we can afford our young clients this opportunity.

CHAPTER SUMMARY

In this chapter, we have considered:

- how a play journal builds into a resource for counsellors – it encourages reflection, gathering of ideas and information and a way to understand play in counselling
- using directed and non-directed play and the reasons counsellors might choose each method or a combination of both

- how different modalities use play and the limitations (e.g. time) that will influence a counsellor's way of playing in counselling
- the physical environment of counselling and how lack of a 'playroom' changes the type of play that can be offered
- play that needs no equipment and play that needs simple, portable equipment only
- counsellors' play kits, how counsellors include play and what informs the choices they make.

REFERENCES

Adler-Tapia, R. (2012) *Child Psychotherapy: Integrating Developmental Theory into Clinical Practice*. New York: Springer.
Angelou, M. (2010) *I Know Why the Caged Bird Sings*. Audio book. Hachette Digital.
Axline, V. (1989) *Play Therapy*. London: Longman.
Bolton, G., Howlett, S., Lago, C. and Wright, J.K. (eds) (2004) *Writing Cures: An Introductory Handbook of Writing in Counselling and Therapy*. Hove: Brunner-Routledge.
Carey, L. (2008) *Sandplay Therapy with Children and Families*. London: Rowman & Littlefield.
Dowsett, G. (2009) *A Toolkit for Developing Emotional Intelligence*. Fishguard, Pembrokeshire: Theatr Fforwm Cymru.
Geldard, K. and Geldard, D. (2008) *Counselling Children: A Practical Introduction*, 3rd edn. London: Sage.
Geldard, K., Geldard, D. and Yin Foo, R. (2013) *Counselling Children*, 4th edn. London: Sage.
Grunwell, E. (2009) *The Freedom Writer's Diary: How a Teacher and 150 Teens Used Writing to Change the World Around Them*. New York: Broadway Books.
Hopper, L. (2007) *Counselling and Psychotherapy with Children and Adolescents*. Basingstoke: Palgrave MacMillan.
Landreth, G. (2012) *Play Therapy: The Art of Relationship*. New York: Taylor & Francis.
McMahon, L. (2005) *Handbook of Play Therapy*. New York: Taylor & Francis.
Mortola, P. (2006) *Windowframes: Learning the Art of Gestalt Play Therapy the Oaklander Way*. Santa Cruz, CA: The Gestalt Press.
Rosen, K. (2009) *Saved by a Poem*. Carlsbad, CA: Hay House.

8

USING SUPERVISION SKILFULLY

INTRODUCTION

In this chapter, supervision of children and young people's counsellors is explored.

Supervision needs to be concerned with counsellors' well-being and not with the client's issues alone. If there are personal issues that affect our work, then supervision is an appropriate place to discuss them.

This chapter aims to help supervisees improve participation in supervision. The Hawkins and Shohet (2007) model offers three areas that need to be covered in supervision: Managerial, Educative and Restorative. This process model of supervision will be applied to the specific issues that arise for counsellors of children and young people. Legal and ethical issues raised in previous chapters can usefully form a basis for supervision, and can be referred to when appropriate.

The BACP now asks for the supervisor's experience with children and young people when accrediting counsellors specifically in this area of counselling. There is recognition of particular skills that are required in a supervisor when clients are young. It is a concern that not all supervisors are aware of the different knowledge and abilities needed when supervising those counselling young clients. Occasionally, a young client can be at risk when the need to act to protect them is missed in supervision. Skilful means at all levels of intervention, including supervision, are needed as this is in the best interests of vulnerable young clients.

Those counselling children and young people need to use supervision wisely, finding a skilful path, gradually growing in confidence and discussing experiences openly. We need to develop our 'internal' supervisor (Henderson and Bailey 2009), and recognise when to consult appropriately with our supervisor outside of regular supervision appointments.

For some counsellors experienced with children and young people, the right time will come to train as supervisors. Supervision courses also need to offer modules specifically designed for learning to supervise counsellors working with children and young people. The idea that supervision designed for counsellors working with adults is suitable for those counselling young clients is one that needs challenging. This chapter seeks to outline a model for children and young people counsellor supervision.

We will examine:

- preparing for supervision
- the differences between the way experienced counsellors and those newly qualified or on placement with children and young people use one-to-one supervision
- good practice – do's and don'ts for individual supervision
- managing time, relationships with other professionals, the pressures of 'paperwork' and administration
- group supervision, boundaries and learning and sharing in a reflective space, including creative activity
- the shape of the supervision process – Managerial, Educative and Restorative processes applied to children and young people's counselling
- using supervision skilfully when we have become over-involved with a young client
- the 'hard to talk about' issues; when we feel we haven't acted well with a young client or with a context issue
- prioritising – recognising issues that need to be more deeply explored
- encouraging mindful self-care and what this entails
- managing the 'caseload', particularly for counsellors with many young clients
- parallel process and how to talk about this in supervision
- celebrating success.

PREPARING FOR SUPERVISION

The type of preparation we choose to make before a supervision session will, in part, depend on our learning style (Honey and Mumford 2006). Those with a reflective learning style may want to take time to go through all their cases well before supervision. Pragmatists will be organised and looking for solutions, theorists will want to explore the theoretical background to their practice and experiential supervisees will want to 'go with the flow', using supervision in an intuitive and spontaneous way. Most of us will combine some of these styles and this will influence the way we prepare.

Unless our supervisor is unusually prescriptive, we will have a say in what we bring to supervision and how we present it. This flexibility asks of supervisees that we give thought to what needs to be included in our supervision. Unless we are students on placement or have a small caseload, we will probably not be speaking about every client we have counselled in each supervision session.

So what skills can we bring to preparation for supervision that will enable best use of the time available? In the BACP information sheet entitled 'How much supervision should I have?' we are reminded that:

Supervision within counselling is based on a 'developmental' rather than a 'deficiency' model of the person. In other words, counselling supervision is not about 'policing', where the emphasis is solely on 'checking up' on you. Instead, the aim is to develop a relationship in which your supervisor is regarded as a trusted colleague who can help you to reflect on all dimensions of your practice and, through that process, to develop your counselling role. (BACP 2008: 1)

With this in mind, we can approach supervision in a manner that means we are working together collaboratively. This can be especially relevant when the clients are children and young people as we can easily become influenced by the general atmosphere of 'checking' and 'monitoring' that often exists within children's services. We, in our role as counsellors, will be subject to checks to see if we have any criminal convictions that would bar us from working with children. Whilst these are necessary precautions, it is useful to counterbalance these requirements with values of trust and mutual respect. Being a 'trusted colleague' means that responsibility exists for both supervisor and supervisee to ensure that supervision is working well.

Assuming you are either in individual supervision or in a small group, you should have enough time to present clients and issues that you need to ask questions about or get support and clarification with. The minimum requirement of 1.5 hours a month of personal time in supervision is only enough if you have a light caseload. For those who have clients numbering around 80 per month, then supervision of 3 hours per month is likely to be needed. Time to talk with line managers or other supportive colleagues is useful but does not replace time in supervision.

If supervision takes place monthly, it is helpful to prepare in this way:

- Review the month. A great deal can happen in a month and it is easy for important issues that took place weeks ago to be overlooked.
- Are there clients who have concerned you each time you counselled them?
- Are there issues in your place of counselling that have consistently been difficult to resolve?
- Are there events in your personal life that are impacting on your practice?
- Make a note of these and roughly the amount of time you want to allocate to each of them.
- Decide what you must include, may include and what it would be nice to include in supervision.
- When you arrive at supervision, you may want to check in and talk about how you are right in that moment. Sometimes an event that has happened just before supervision becomes so insistent to be spoken of that this needs to be given time, though it might not be the most important aspect of that month's supervision. Examples of this are given below.

CASE EXAMPLE: ONE-TO-ONE SUPERVISION WITH AN EXPERIENCED COUNSELLOR

Janice has 2 hours of individual supervision provided by her employers each month; she works for four days per week in a secondary school with 1500 pupils. Janice very rarely contacts her supervisor between monthly sessions although she knows this option exists and has the mobile phone number of her supervisor. Janice has been in her post for three years and is well aware of how to manage liaison with staff at the school, disclosures and child protection procedures, as well as making sure her clients are given time and attention appropriately. The main, regular challenge for Janice is managing the amount of administration and paperwork that comes with a caseload of up to 20 clients per week.

Janice's agenda for supervision is as follows:

- Garth has witnessed domestic violence and there is a multi-agency meeting next week to which Janice has been invited. She is expected to report Garth's progress and give her opinion as to whether her young client is at risk. Janice is concerned about maintaining Garth's confidentiality and doing her best to explain the feelings of her client at the same time. Janice has experienced this type of meeting before and wants to discuss it in supervision (see Chapter 5 on multi-agency meetings).

- Janice has recently had to change the room she counsels in. This has been difficult as the new room, although pleasant, opens directly on to a busy corridor and young clients are seen entering and leaving. Some of Janice's clients have been commenting on the fact that they have seen others they know entering and leaving the counselling room. Janice, of course, never comments or enters into conversation about other clients. She is feeling unsure about how to manage this new room. Should she ask to be moved again or are there ways to ease the problems associated with the room?

- Recently, the agency Janice counsels for has asked her to enter some statistical information electronically via a secure system. Janice, along with some other counsellors employed by the same agency, is having difficulty with the new administrative demands. The demands of 'admin' are very time consuming at a busy time of year. Janice wants to talk about how best to manage this and to just 'let off steam' at the complications caused by activities quite remote from client work itself.

- Finally, hours before Janice was due to arrive for supervision, her car broke down, meaning she was late for work and missed seeing a client whom she had planned to see at 9.15 that morning. Janice feels concerned about her busy week and fitting in clients when unexpected events like this occur.

Questions to consider:

- Janice has 2 hours of supervision – how can she best manage the time available?
- Which of the above issues do you think she should prioritise in supervision?
- Is there anything her supervisor might want to discuss that is not on Janice's initial agenda?

The supervisor's role with an experienced counsellor

Janice's supervisor recognises the level of skill and experience in her work and wants to encourage her to use supervision in a way that is best. There is a recognition on the supervisor's part that it is important to keep awareness of any aspects of Janice's work that may have been missed and to hold Janice's need to be restored by supervision, recognising Janice might not prioritise this herself.

CASE EXAMPLE: A COUNSELLOR ON PLACEMENT IN A SCHOOL COMES TO SUPERVISION

Pete is a trainee counsellor on placement in a secondary school. He has teaching experience and wants to change his career to become a counsellor. He is in his second year of training as a counsellor and his supervisor needs to write a report about him in order to fulfil the requirements of his training course. Pete is also required to discuss all of his clients in supervision.

For Pete, there are issues about his role as a counsellor rather than a teacher that he needs to discuss in supervision. Whilst he is very keen to be a counsellor, he finds it strange at times to be in a confidential, individual relationship with children in school. He explains to his supervisor that the school staff feel reassured that he has a teaching qualification and want to talk to him about the difficulties they are finding with the children who have been referred to counselling. Pete recognises the pressures teachers are under and wants to offer support to them without disclosing anything from the counselling sessions.

Pete has 1.5 hours of supervision allocated to him each month. There is also a requirement for him to be in contact with his supervisor fortnightly as a trainee counsellor. He and his supervisor have decided on a 15-minute phone call and

(Continued)

(Continued)

a meeting for 1.25 hours each month. With four clients and the context issues he wants to bring to supervision, he feels under pressure to fit everything into his allocated supervision time.

The 15-minute phone call this month was taken up with Pete's worries about whether one young client's issues require a disclosure or not. Pete has seen this client once more since the phone call with his supervisor and needs to update on the situation with the client during this session.

Pete arrives at supervision looking a bit flustered and saying that he doesn't know how he is going to fit everything in. His supervisor reminds him that they had agreed to discuss the report that needs to be written for his training course in this supervision session. Pete expresses concern that his clients might not get enough 'air time' if the report is given priority.

Questions to consider:

- How does Pete manage his time in supervision?
- How can his supervisor help him to prioritise?

Answers to the above questions are addressed in the following good practice do's and don'ts.

ONE-TO-ONE SUPERVISION — GOOD PRACTICE DO'S AND DON'TS

- Do think about the overall time you have available in supervision and roughly map out how many minutes you have for each issue.
- Do consider your clients overall — are there 'themes' that you can cover in supervision? Perhaps more than one client with similar or comparable issues can be given attention by discussing, for example, 'bullying' or 'divorce and separation in the family'.
- Do allow time to bring personal issues to supervision that may impact on your ability to counsel young clients. Sometimes getting something 'off your chest' in supervision makes your caseload feel more manageable.
- Do discuss context issues in your place of work that are giving cause for concern. You may need to decide on a course of action with your supervisor and keep in contact with them as the situation progresses to ensure the safety of young clients.
- Do consider finding ways to extend your supervision time if you regularly feel pressurised or rushed. Sometimes this involves talking to your placement, agency or employer about them giving you more time in supervision. Some supervisees pay for extra time with their supervisor. Whilst this may not be ideal, if your agency is in the voluntary sector, financial pressures may mean that this is the best solution available.

- Do talk with your supervisor about how the supervisory relationship is working for you. You may find that your supervisor has had a very different kind of training or has differing beliefs about counselling. It is best to discuss any differences that arise.

- Do remember that whilst your supervisor may be more experienced than you, they are not automatically more knowledgeable or correct on every issue. You will need to discuss matters very thoroughly if your supervisor questions your practice and you believe you have acted in accordance with your training and ethical principles.

- Do ensure you aim for collaboration, problem solving and finding the best outcomes for your clients.

- Don't become defensive in supervision. An open mind and a sense of exploration together are part of good practice in the supervision process.

- Don't always wait for your appointment time. If something seriously concerns you in your practice, speak to your supervisor as soon as possible.

- Do find a supervisor who is contactable for urgent cases at short notice and has locum cover available if they are away or on leave. This access to supervision between monthly sessions is vital when clients are children and young people, as the need to act on behalf of clients is more frequent.

- Do use other forms of contact than 'face to face' if you need to due to long travelling distances or other commitments. The majority of the report that Pete, in the case study above, needs for his course can be completed online and emailed, for example, allowing client issues to be prioritised. The telephone call mid-month is very helpful for Pete and using Skype is also an acceptable method of supervision contact.

- Don't try to manage without supervision because you are very busy or have missed an appointment through ill health.

- Do pay attention to your level of supervision and if there is not enough time or if there is something in the supervisory relationship that is not working for you, address this as soon as possible with your supervisor.

GROUP SUPERVISION

The BACP has a calculation that in a group of two, three or four members, half the time the group runs for can be considered as personal supervision by each member. This means that in a monthly three-hour supervision group with four members, each member can claim an hour-and-a-half of individual supervision time. Groups with five or more members need to divide the length of supervision by the number of supervisees present. In supervision groups with five members that take place monthly for three hours, each member can claim 36 minutes of personal supervision time.

The BACP calculation of group supervision time means that some organisations offer their counsellors groups with four members for 3 hours each month to meet the recommended minimum.

If counsellors are working with young clients on placement or on a part-time basis for one or two days per week, the supervision group alone may work well. Groups have the advantage of offering the opportunity to hear other people's casework and learning to respond to others in the group, as well as noticing how the supervisor gives guidance and support or asks questions in each case.

If, however, we have many young clients to discuss, the group will probably not be enough. It is also possible to hide in a supervision group and appear to have few needs when in fact aspects of our client work are not being supervised. Ideally, every supervisee needs plenty of time to review and process their counselling and this time is for and on behalf of our clients as well as for us.

Proctor (2008) gives us the idea that agreements are 'friends' in group supervision:

- First, we have non-negotiable boundaries such as confidentiality and monitoring. Here, we learn that ethical considerations, such as ethical issues with safety implications for young clients, *must* be brought to supervision.

- Next is the group working agreement with 'ground rules' which defines the group's relationship with 'fairness and trust' and gives permission to opt out. Here, we also discuss challenge and risk and become close to others in a supervision group.

- Third, there is a session agenda. This includes the opportunity for brief personal check-ins, time to build an agenda, presenting of clients and a review at the end.

- Finally, there is the 'heart' of the supervision group – the reflective space where learning and change take place. In this 'mini contract' in the centre of a supervision group, the supervisee identifies their own present state. All the other parts of the agreement allow this reflection to take place.

- When the group is for supervising children and young people's counselling, particular emphasis can be put on learning about and sharing resources and identifying common themes that most counsellors are managing. For example, the following issues are likely to be raised frequently in the group:

    o suitable rooms for counselling young clients
    o being asked to share information in meetings
    o liaising with adults to get young clients into counselling
    o young clients' language and use of terminology
    o internet use
    o young clients on prescription medication
    o mental health diagnoses and engaging with child and adolescent mental health services
    o managing non-attendance and waiting lists.

These are important topics to discuss, but they can overwhelm the group and mean that the heart of the matter, the reflective space, gets minimised or neglected. We need to ensure that practical concerns do not become everything in group supervision of children and young people's counselling.

Creativity, fun and laughter can all be part of the supervision group. An activity that offers learning in a creative way and can then be adapted for use with young clients is outlined below:

Activity: Collage of a client

Bring in old magazines, blank paper and sticks of glue.

1. In the group, each member has five minutes to tear out pictures or words that will illustrate a young client they are counselling. This is best done quickly and without too much planning.
2. Once the five minutes is up, everyone looks at each other's collage. Nothing is said at this stage as quiet observation takes place.
3. Each member holds up their collage and other members of the group say what they notice. The person who made the collage just listens.
4. Once everyone has received feedback on their collage, there is an opportunity to talk about what it was like to make the collage and hear how others found it.
5. An extension of this exercise would be an in-depth exploration of a client and the relationship with their counsellor using insights gained from the collage. Counsellors can use this type of activity with young clients and there is an example of this in Chapter 7.

THE SHAPE OF SUPERVISION: MANAGERIAL, EDUCATIVE AND RESTORATIVE

Hawkins and Shohet (2007) have suggested that supervision can be divided into three sections: Managerial, Educative and Restorative. This is useful to supervision where the clients are children and young people. Applying this model helps to ensure that nothing important is missed out of the supervision process:

- The Managerial or 'Normative' aspect of supervision offers an opportunity for the supervisor and supervisee to focus on matters that ensure safe, competent practice is taking place.
- The Educative aspect is where new learning takes place, either through the supervisor passing on their knowledge, skills and experience or from researching a matter that arises from client work.
- The Restorative aspect is usually included last of the three, yet is probably most crucial in enabling safe practice with children and young people. Hawkins and Shohet (2007) offer the analogy of coal miners' 'pit head time'. As part of their working day, miners won the right to wash off the grime of their work in the coal

mine before going home. A similar and comparable process happens to counsellors and therapists in the way we absorb the problems and issues of our clients into ourselves. The term 'mirror neurons' (Rothschild 1993) is used to explain that it is now recognised that by opening ourselves up to deep empathy and connection with our clients, we actually change ourselves bodily and become, at least momentarily, more like our clients. Restorative processes in supervision offer the opportunity to 'wash off' anything that has stuck to us from our clients. Whilst it is important that we are able to closely relate to our clients' experiences, if we cannot return to ourselves, replenish and restore, then exhaustion and fatigue will quickly follow. Our ability to make use of the restorative part of supervision is crucial to good practice.

In the following case example, these three aspects of supervision are highlighted.

CASE EXAMPLE: CONCERNS ABOUT YOUR OWN COMPETENCY

Your client is a 15-year-old boy who is having 'demonic' visions after substance misuse. He is sent to see you by his head of year at school because of his inability to concentrate in class. He seems to be in a world of his own and you sense that you are not connecting with him. You feel relieved at the end of the session with him but are left with an upsetting memory of what he is 'seeing'. In supervision, your supervisor notices how fearful you look as you speak of counselling this client.

Skills for supervision

Managerial considerations

- Is safe practice taking place?
- Are you 'out of your depth' with this particular client?
- Does the client need to be referred to more specialised help and, if so, what is available in your area? (Many specialist substance misuse agencies exist and some can come into schools and see young people.)

Educative considerations

- What do you know about the particular issues that are involved in this case? There may be a lack of knowledge about and a need for education and training on:
  - substance misuse and young people
  - recognising the onset of mental health conditions in teenagers
  - psychosis that begins in teenage years.

There are simple and effective ways to learn more about your client's condition. Local and national agencies will have leaflets and information online. Issues can be raised in supervision and followed up through research and training opportunities. It may be the first time you have met a client like this. Feelings of being scared of demonic visions and a client losing touch with reality can be vastly reduced once knowledge, training and support are in place. This learning will take time and it may be necessary for your supervisor to support you with this client. It is important to note that there should be no blame or criticism because there is a lack of knowledge. We cannot be 'experts' in every field and need to recognise what we don't know and those we cannot help in counselling.

Restorative considerations

It may be an upsetting and frightening moment for you to realise you cannot reach this young person who is lost in his world of demons. You might also be aware that other counsellors are not scared or upset by this type of case and then blame yourself for weakness or feel incompetent because it is affecting you. Alternatively, you might blame this young client, thinking he has 'brought his problem on himself' or 'caused unnecessary problems for his family and school'. In either of these reactions, there has been a loss of balance, perhaps picking up on the client's disturbance and feeling disturbed by them. A counter-transference may be in operation where you have taken on the role of a parent or other critical person, feeling afraid and 'helpless' rather than remaining in a counselling role. If something from this client has 'stuck' to you, supervision is the place to explore and release this.

It is important for your supervisor to be able to both support and challenge you in this circumstance. Your supervisor needs to connect with you as the focus is now on restoring you and not directly on your client. In counselling, *we* are the 'tool' of our trade. If a tradesperson does not take time to check their equipment is working properly, they cannot do their work. If we do not address the impact of young clients upon us, accepting that some will have a significant effect on the quality of our practice, then we are missing out on a vital part of supervision.

WHEN WE THINK WE HAVEN'T ACTED WELL OR HAVE GOT IT WRONG

Supervision is a good time to sort out difficulties that arise when counselling children and young people. Our profession's mandatory supervision requirement brings a wonderful opportunity to improve practice and continuously develop into a more skilful practitioner.

If we think that we have made a mistake whilst counselling, the best approach is to consider the reality of the situation in supervision. How is it best to do this?

Being a skilful supervisee involves:

- bringing issues to supervision with clarity and at a good time
- accurate recall of what happened, bringing the 'whole picture' to supervision

- ◆ not blaming ourselves or others for problems that arise in practice – it is not a question of who is at fault, rather about gaining understanding and looking for the best way forward (see Chapter 6 on resolving ethical dilemmas)

- ◆ recognising there may be angry feelings in us, in our clients and in their families – whilst it is understandable when we hear stories of abuse of children to be angry with the abusers, reacting from a place of anger can cause more problems than it solves

- ◆ being prepared to reflect on our practice in a calm and considered manner

- ◆ accepting that sometimes we will feel emotional in supervision and that this is part of the way of managing to witness and be present with the distressing circumstances of young clients' lives.

Issues that we are not aware of

Occasionally, supervisors pick up on issues that we are not aware of. Anyone can, occasionally, make a real, tangible mistake in counselling that needs sorting out. Very experienced and excellent practitioners sometimes get it wrong. What is important is to learn from mistakes and minimise their impact on clients. Commonly, mistakes come about from caring too much rather than too little. One of the hardest aspects of counselling children and young people is accepting our own limitations and knowing that we do not have a magic potion that will make a child or young person's life better. Some counsellors who start working with children and young people cannot manage witnessing the depth of pain of a suffering youngster and opt for counselling adults. Great resilience is required and an acceptance that suffering exists for so many children and young people – it is not our fault that we cannot cure it.

Encouraging mindful self-care in supervision to help prevent mistakes and 'burn-out'

The self-care aspect of supervision is not a nice 'add-on'. I once heard a trainer teaching self-care say to a group 'don't tell me you are going have a bath or a glass of wine'. I knew exactly what she meant. Whilst these may be useful, relaxing activities to help switch off from the working day, counsellors of children and young people require a much deeper understanding of self-care.

The realities of children's and young people's lives *will* affect us sometimes. We need to develop whole-life strategies that will continuously rebuild our resilience and supervision needs to be part of the strategy. Learning to be mindful in everyday life is an example of a whole of life practice that can sustain us in our work. If our supervision is not restorative, not part of the self-care that enables us to return to being alongside young clients who are suffering, then it is not working properly.

MINDFUL MOMENT: CONTACTING YOUR 'INNER SUPERVISOR'

Find a quiet place to sit where you won't be interrupted. Sit in an upright position, giving yourself time just to breathe. When you are ready, close your eyes and bring to mind your 'inner supervisor'. This is a being who embodies your wisdom and knowing. They may look like you or be entirely different from you. They may be in a room that is significant or outside in nature.

Notice the qualities of this being. Ask them if they have any information they would like to offer you. Take time to converse with your inner supervisor or sit in silence, sensing their presence. When you have discovered all you want to for now, say farewell, knowing that this 'inner supervisor' is available to you when needed. Open your eyes and take a moment to adjust to everyday life.

Make notes of what has happened in this practice and share any insights with trusted colleagues or your supervisor. You may find that this type of activity develops your intuitive abilities and gives you access to that part of you that knows what is best. Always check any insights found in this way with your supervisor before acting on them.

Common difficulties that can be addressed in supervision

1 Giving too much information

Breaches of confidentiality can occur when we have been asked a question and given too much information in response. Whilst presenting a client in supervision, a counsellor may say, 'I discussed what the client said with their teacher or parent'. When their supervisor then asks 'did you have your client's permission to talk about that?', sometimes the answer is no or a hasty response like 'I don't think this client would mind'. In this case, the counsellor in question may have overstepped the boundary of confidentiality, even though they felt they were acting in their young client's best interests. This situation occurs quite frequently because children and young people have fewer rights to confidentiality and autonomy than adults. Adults assume that counsellors will talk to them about a client. There may be expectations from the organisations who employ us that we will share information. This expectation can directly contradict the confidential relationship we have with our young client (Copeland 2013).

It is often because we are kind, caring people that we give away too much information. It can be very awkward to explain why we are not talking about our client's issues to a concerned parent or teacher. Good practice in responding to difficult questions is given in Chapter 5 on confidentiality.

As we have discovered in earlier chapters, respecting young clients' right to privacy is vital in most situations and it is a betrayal of trust to just talk about a confidential disclosure unthinkingly to adults.

Knowing too much has been said Sometimes a counsellor will know they have said too much in response to a question or in a meeting, regret it and want to discuss this in supervision. It is often best to work out how to let the young client know that this breach of their confidence has taken place. Mostly, problems arising from this can be easily resolved with the client and do not materially affect the counselling relationship.

Occasionally though, the consequences of letting something 'slip' are very great, so practising suitable replies to concerned adults is helpful to prevent getting caught up in sharing too much information.

Considering the way that a breach of confidentiality came about is a matter that needs to be brought to supervision. Reasons why counsellors feel they mistakenly talked to adults about a child need to be examined and clarified.

When parents are paying for counselling and are concerned and upset about their child, it is hard for them to understand why you don't tell them everything the child has said. Teachers and other professionals may assume a right to know what is happening in counselling. Supervision is the best place to explore good practice in these situations.

Feeling shame Counsellors may feel ashamed or upset, thinking they have made a serious mistake. A productive relationship between supervisor and supervisee is one where there can be learning from mistakes, ensuring that any consequences are addressed and there is an adult-to-adult alliance between supervisee and supervisor.

2 Becoming over-involved with a client

Over-involvement can happen with a client of any age. The wish to act on behalf of a younger client becomes more pressing because of children and young people's lack of power to change their own lives. Counsellors need to learn to pick up on the signs that they have become too involved and openly discuss this in supervision.

Noticing rescuing behaviour Supervisors too should notice if a counsellor has veered into attempting to rescue a child or young person from their life situation. It can be deeply distressing to not be able to change a young client's life. It has been explained in earlier chapters how and when counsellors need to act to help those whose life situations are abusive or neglectful. Supervision is the place where checking and confirming actions that need to be taken can be done.

Noticing sexual feelings Flirtatious behaviour from a child or young person in counselling can be challenging. What do you do if a young person feels attracted to you or imagines they have 'fallen in love' with you? What do you do if you feel flattered or drawn towards a young client who is behaving in a sexual manner in counselling? It is necessary to bring all issues concerning sexuality to supervision (Corey et al. 2011: 301).

Emerging sexuality is one of the main concerns of adolescence and counsellors have a unique opportunity to offer a clear, straightforward, adult, non-judgemental response to young people who need to talk about sex. There are many young clients in counselling who have been sexually abused or who are concerned about their partnerships and their sexual feelings.

If a counsellor senses a young client is sexually attracted to them or if a counsellor experiences feelings of attraction for their client, this must be discussed with their supervisor. It is *never* appropriate to respond to a young client's sexual behaviour or feelings of attraction by flirting with them. It may be necessary to reiterate the safety boundaries of counselling during supervision.

Counsellors know how to act safely and ethically with young people, but, when sexual feelings are present, may become embarrassed or fearful. Getting support in this situation is vital. Counselling can then help young people establish healthy sexual boundaries without feeling judged or rejected.

3 Stepping into the role of a family member

It is common for counsellors to step into a parental role with young clients. In supervision, we can talk about our feelings of wanting to take a young client home with us. It is a compassionate, human response to want to save young people from aggressive or neglectful parenting. We can remind ourselves to take a step back from our need to be a 'nurturing angel' or a 'lone ranger' when we come to supervision. Getting an overview of the whole situation can help us act with more clarity and sensitivity in counselling.

Sometimes, however, counsellors may step into the role of a critical parent and judge a client. Supervision is useful for recognising this and why it may be happening.

We may also form an alliance with a family member we have never met but feel great sympathy for.

CASE EXAMPLE: JO JUDGES HER CLIENT, KIM

Jo counsels in a youth centre and comes to supervision wanting to talk about feelings of being 'cross' with a client, Kim. Kim is 15 and her mother has had a new baby recently. The baby doesn't sleep well. Kim is over-tired and getting low marks at school because the baby is awake at night and its crying wakes Kim up. There are no lifts to town for Kim at the moment as her mum and step-dad are pre-occupied with the new baby. Kim is angry and resentful at being asked to do more at home.

As Jo describes the situation in supervision, there is an edge in her voice. She says, 'oh, Kim is so hard done by! She complains that she has to wash up more often'! Jo's supervisor looks at her with a slightly puzzled expression and asks Jo what happens to her when she hears Kim complaining. Jo goes quiet for

(Continued)

(Continued)

a moment and feels a little fed up that her supervisor is not joining her in thinking of Kim as a stroppy teenager who wants everything her own way. Jo muses on how annoying Kim is and thinks that perhaps she is wasting supervision time in talking about Kim as the issues in this case are 'trivial' in comparison to those of some other clients.

Jo looks up and her supervisor asks: 'Does Kim remind you of anyone'? Jo looks surprised and says, 'Well, actually she reminds me of my older sister who always thought I was in the way'. The supervisor waits and Jo begins to speak of her sister, much older than her, who was made to take care of Jo. Jo's sister had felt resentment and had been nasty and bullied Jo at times. 'It wasn't my fault but she took it out on me', Jo says to her supervisor.

As the supervision progresses, Jo begins to understand how the similarities between her client and her own older sister are affecting the way she counsels in this case. Jo has residual feelings of being angry at the way her sister treated her and this is being expressed in her being fed up and unable to empathise with Kim. Eventually, Jo begins to recognise some differences between Kim and her own sister and even sees the funny side of her vehement complaining about Kim.

In supervision, there is an opportunity to more fully recognise how our own family situation, past or present, may influence our ability to counsel a particular client. It is not a question of trying to avoid this influence, rather it's about becoming more skilled in recognising where and when we are vulnerable as counsellors. If there were repeated events of the kind that have arisen when counselling Kim, a supervisor might suggest personal counselling for Jo as further support for her.

Only in very extreme and occasional circumstances would a supervisor insist that a counsellor stops practising, but this route could be taken if there was a clear sense that a counsellor was not practising safely and competently. The needs of a child or young person who is in counselling must be the first priority, so if a supervisor recognises a significant problem then action must be taken to keep a young client safe.

Gaining insight The important element here is that Jo has gained insight into her own bias that has been stimulated by her client, Kim. This insight will most probably be enough for Jo to release the projection she had placed on Kim and begin to be able to empathise with her. The supervisor would need to check in the following supervision session that changes had been made in the counselling and that now there is a more client-centred approach, rather than a critical, judgemental one in this counselling relationship.

Making mistakes is part of being human. There is pressure to never get anything wrong when the client is a vulnerable child or young person. If mistakes are brought to supervision, learning and insight can come from courageously and thoroughly investigating them. The therapeutic alliance that was identified in Chapter 1 is, ideally, mirrored in the supervisory alliance. A sense of working through issues together is vital in supervision.

Parallel process

Understanding the nature of parallel process is very useful in the supervision of children and young people's counselling. Parallel process is present when a counsellor brings to mind a particular client in supervision and they start to speak and act in ways that show characteristics of that client. If parallel process is unrecognised, the supervisor, in turn, may begin to respond in ways that are similar to how the counsellor responded to that client.

CASE EXAMPLE: RALPH

Ralph is a 12-year-old who is often confused and his counsellor finds it difficult to understand what he is saying as he 'mumbles' and his speech is disjointed. Ralph's counsellor, Sonia, decides to bring Ralph to supervision.

Sonia begins to talk about Ralph in supervision. Sonia's speech becomes indistinct and she stops and starts speaking, just like Ralph, losing the thread of what she is saying. Her supervisor begins to feel confused and it becomes harder and harder to maintain good communication in supervision.

If this parallel process goes unrecognised, then it can be misinterpreted as a confused counsellor in supervision. One way to know that parallel process is happening is to change the subject under discussion. When Ralph is no longer being 'presented' in supervision, then the whole atmosphere changes and communication flows once again.

Supervisors can 'pick up' on parallel process and comment on it. This is very helpful and sometimes has the quality of 'breaking a spell', enabling a different kind of discussion about a client to take place. There can be great benefit in parallel process taking place in supervision. It is not a mistake, but it can present moments of confusion or difficulty that require us to consider what is happening in supervision in another way.

To help with considering the different aspects of communication in supervision, we can refer to Hawkins and Shohet's 'seven-eyed' model (Wilmot 2012). This model recognises that a counsellor talking about their client is just one of seven modes of communication between supervisor and supervisee. As we move through 'bringing' our young client into supervision, we consider our relationship with that client and what our interventions were. We then move deeper into considering how we see our clients, how they see us and the transferences that are taking place.

We go on through the 'eyes' to consider the nature of the relationship between supervisor and supervisee and how this 'mirrors' relationships in counselling. Finally, we take into account the 'waters we are swimming in' (Wilmot 2012) – those context issues that may need examination in our counselling. How we manage relationships with colleagues within any organisation where we counsel is a key issue in supervision (Copeland 2013).

Feeling stuck

Useful activities in supervision that help if we are 'stuck' or need to gain insight include the following:

- Become your client – take a few minutes to speak 'as' the client in supervision.
- Imagine you are on a desert island with your client. Where would you both be on the island? How are you relating to each other?
- Become your client whilst your supervisor plays the role of an interviewer from school or college who is writing about the counselling service and wants to know what you think of counselling.

Your supervisor can ask simple questions: Why do you go to counselling? What do you like? What don't you like?

After this activity, de-role by speaking about your own life in the present. Becoming the client not only gives insight, it can have a prolonged influence if the exercise is not completed by actively 'letting go' of it.

CELEBRATING SUCCESS

A vital part of supervision in children and young people's counselling is to celebrate success and talk about what has gone well. Statistical information is showing how much counselling services are valued by children and young people. Counsellors in this field have reason to celebrate at times about the heart-warming successes that young clients achieve through coming to counselling.

Whether it is the ability to talk to a parent or teacher in a new way; to understand that they are not to blame for difficult life circumstances when they have been blamed and victimised; to sleep, eat or simply communicate in a way they have not been able to before coming to counselling – all these achievements can be celebrated. Bringing successes to supervision and celebrating them is as important as bringing difficulties, as it helps to maintain resilience.

CHAPTER SUMMARY

Supervision is vital for all counselling and therapeutic work. There is a need to:

- have access to our supervisor between monthly sessions
- understand how clients can affect us and unravel any difficulties in supervision

- recognise if we are not getting enough supervision of the kind we need
- take an active and collaborative part in supervision and think of our supervisor as a 'trusted colleague'
- be courageous in supervision, looking deeply at ourselves, our motivations and fears
- celebrate success, recognising we are part of a team of people whose concern is the well-being of all children and young people.

REFERENCES

British Association for Counselling and Psychotherapy (BACP) (2008) Information Sheet S1: 'How much supervision should I have?' Lutterworth: BACP.

Copeland, S. (2013) *Counselling Supervision in Organisations: Professional and Ethical Dilemmas Explored*. Hove: Routledge.

Corey, G., Corey, M.S. and Callahan, P. (2011) *Issues and Ethics in the Helping Professions*. Pacific Grove, CA: Brooks Cole/Cengage Learning.

Hawkins, P. and Shohet, R. (2007) *Supervision in the Helping Professions*, 3rd edn. Maidenhead: McGraw-Hill International.

Henderson, P. and Bailey, C. (2009) 'The internal supervisor: developing the witness within', in P. Henderson, P. (ed.), *Supervisor Training: Issues and Approaches*. London: Karnac Books, pp. 93–107.

Honey, P. and Mumford, A. (2006) *Learning Styles Questionnaire*. Maidenhead: P. Honey Publications.

Proctor, B. (2008) *Group Supervison: A Guide to Creative Practice*. London: Sage.

Rothschild, B. (1993) Transference and Countertransference: A Common Sense Perspective. Available at: www.toddlertime.com/mh/terms/countertransference-transference-2.htm

Wilmot, J. (2012) Hawkins and Shohet's Seven-eyed Model of Supervision. Available at: http://youtu.be/JJwhpz8NSV0

INDEX

abuse, 130, 132–135
acceptance, 74
active listening, 82
adults. *See* parents and carers
advocacy, 38–39
age-appropriateness, 9–10, 23–24, 27
agreements, 116–119
All Wales Child Protection Procedures, 130
analogies, 99–100
Angelou, M., 160
anger management, 89
anonymity, 160
assessment
  dilemmas in, 29–31
  forms for, 31–35
  process of, 35–40
  role of adults in, 40–51
attachment theory, 22, 85, 91
autonomy, 116, 122, 124
Axline, V., 95–96, 153

BACP (British Association for Counselling and Psychotherapy)
  Ethical Framework by, 10, 51, 52, 116, 122–129, 131
  on supervision, 165, 166–167, 171
Batmanghelidjh, C., 76
behaviour therapy, 149
beneficence, 10, 116, 122, 124–125
blob tree, 97–98
board games, 159
Bowlby, J., 22, 91
breathing, 159
Brice, A., 65
burn-out, 11, 176
Byron, T., 140

Casemore, R., 129
child ego state, 9
child protection, 116, 119, 130–136
Childline, 140

Children's Act (1989), 113, 115, 130
Children's Legal Centre, 107, 112
Clarke, P., 137
Clywch Report, 137
cognitive-behavioural therapy (CBT), 82, 84–91, 148, 149
communication styles, 54–55
compassion-focused therapy, 90–91
confidentiality
  adults and, 41
  agreements and, 8, 116–119
  assessment and, 35
  beneficence and, 125
  breaches of, 177–178
  disclosure and, 10–11, 18–19
  Gillick competence and, 18, 111–116, 130
  importance of, 104–106
  legal framework and, 111–112
  person-centred counselling and, 98–99
  resilience and, 10–11
congruence, 147
connection, 58–62
consent forms, 107–108
contracts, 38, 116–119
Cooper, M., 34
counselling skills
  connection, 53, 58–62
  developing the relationship, 53, 70–79
  H.E.A.R.O.S., 7–13, 27
  presence, 53, 55–58
  respect, 53, 62–69
  skills in relating, 53, 54–55
counselling with children and young people
  access to, 16, 137
  basic principles and requirements for, 14–16
  theories and, 19–22
  as voluntary, 15–16, 124
counter-transference, 175
creative imagination, 62–69
creative writing, 159–160, 162–163
culture, 71

Index

Daniels, D., 104, 113–114, 130–131
Data Protection Act, 118
directed play, 148, 149
disclosure, 10–11, 18–19, 67–68
diversity, 70–71
drawing, 160

email, 139
emotional abuse, 134–135
emotional literacy, 6–7, 87, 92–94, 157–158
empathy, 9
endings, 78–79
Erikson, E., 20
ethical dilemmas
   BACP Ethical Framework and, 10, 51, 52, 116, 122–129, 131
   child protection and, 116, 119, 130–136
   internet and, 138–141
   introduction to, 121–122
   school counsellors and, 137–138
   See also confidentiality
ethical mindfulness, 122

family photos, 86–87
family trees, 87–88
fantasy, 62–69
feelings. *See* emotional literacy
fibs, 62–69
fidelity, 122, 123, 128–129
Fraser Guidelines, 114
The Freedom Writer's Diary (Grunwell), 160

Gabriel, L., 129
Geldard, D.
   on inner adolescent, 60
   on Maslow, 19
   on play, 148–149, 150–151
   on proactive approach, 96–97
   on respect, 65
Geldard, K.
   on inner adolescent, 60
   on Maslow, 19
   on play, 148–149, 150–151, 159
   on proactive approach, 96–97
   on respect, 65
genograms, 87–88
Gestalt therapy, 96, 148, 152–153
gifts, 126
Gillick competence, 18, 42, 111–116, 130
Green, J., 56
group supervision, 171–173
Grunwell, E., 160

Hawkins, P., 165, 173–174, 181
H.E.A.R.O.S., 7–13, 27
helplines, 49
honesty, 74

Hopper, L., 151
humanistic approaches, 95–99

identity crisis, 20
imaginary superheroes and superheroines, 158–159
immediacy, 75–76
In Treatment (TV series), 109
initial training, 31, 82
inner supervisor, 83
integrative approach, 83–84, 148–149, 150–151
internet, 138–141

Jenkins, P., 104, 113–114, 130–131
jigsaws, 159
Joyce, P., 129
justice, 123, 126–127

Kabat-Zinn, J., 13
Kohlberg, L., 20–21

Landreth, G., 163
language, 71
law and legal framework, 15, 111–112. *See also* Gillick competence
Levine, P., 24–26
lies, 62–69
life stage theory, 20
lifeline, 85–86
Linehan, M., 32
Loesser, F.H., 29
lyrics, 159–160

Maslow, A., 19
metaphors, 99–100
mindful noticing, 58
mindful observation, 152
mindful self-care, 13, 27, 176–177
mindfulness, 13
mirror neurons, 11, 73, 174
money, 126
moral values, 71
Morgan, A., 41, 101
motivational interviewing, 82
multi-agency meetings, 123

narrative therapy, 100–101, 148, 149
neglect, 134–135
no talk therapy, 101
non-directed play, 95–96, 148, 149–150, 151
non-maleficence, 122, 125–126, 128–129
notes, 118

Oaklander, V., 89, 96
one-to-one supervision, 168–171
openness to difference, 12

painting, 160
parallel process, 181–182
parents and carers
   communication with, 17–19, 40–51, 108–110
   confidentiality and, 105, 107
   referral processes and, 40–51
person-centred counselling, 82, 95–99, 148, 153–154
personal counselling, 11
physical abuse, 133
Piaget, J., 20
play
   circumstances of counselling and, 154–157
   client-centred approach and, 95–96, 148, 153–154
   cognitive-behavioural therapy and, 88–89, 148, 149
   Gestalt therapy and, 148, 152–153
   integrative approach and, 148–149, 150–151
   internet and, 139–140
   materials for, 157–163
   narrative therapy and, 148, 149
   psychodynamic approach and, 148, 151–152
   therapeutic value of, 143–144
   trauma and, 24–26
play journals, 145–148
play kits, 160–163
Play Therapy (Axline), 95–96
playing cards, 159
poetry, 159–160
presence, 55–58
privacy, 126
proactive approach, 96–97
Proctor, B., 172
psychodynamic approach, 82, 91–95, 148, 151–152

qualifications, 14
quietness, 77–78

referral procedures, 15–16, 40–51
Reid, H.L., 50
relaxation, 159
religious values, 71
rescuing behaviour, 178
resilience, 10
resistance, 76–77, 82
resource directories, 49–50
respect, 62–69, 109
rights, 15
Rogers, C., 46
Rothschild, B., 11, 73, 74

school counsellors, 137–138
self-care, 13, 27, 176–177

self-directed play, 151
self-disclosure, 94–95
self-harm, 132, 133–134
self-respect, 123, 127–128
sex, 131, 132
sexting, 140
sexual abuse, 132–133
sexual feelings, 178–179
Shohet, R., 165, 173–174, 181
significant harm, 66, 104, 130
Sills, C., 129
social media sites, 139
stories, 159–160, 162–163
Straus, M., 101
style, 71
success, 182
superheroes and superheroines, 158–159
supervision
   assessment and, 47
   BACP Ethical Framework and, 165, 166–167, 171
   difficulties and mistakes addressed in, 175–182
   group supervision, 171–173
   integrative approach and, 83
   lifeline and, 86
   managerial, educative and restorative aspects of, 173–175
   one-to-one supervision, 168–171
   person-centred counselling and, 98
   preparing for, 166–170
   resilience and, 11
   success and, 182
   supervisor's experience and, 117
   tips for, 170–171
systemic counselling, 99–100

tall stories, 62–69
therapeutic alliance, 5–13, 54
thin descriptions, 41
Transactional Analysis (TA), 9, 60–61, 83–84
trauma, 24–26, 27
Twigg, E., 34

under-age sex, 131, 132
United Nations Convention on the Rights of the Child, 113, 115

Weiss, L., 11
Westergaard, J., 26, 50

YP CORE, 32–35

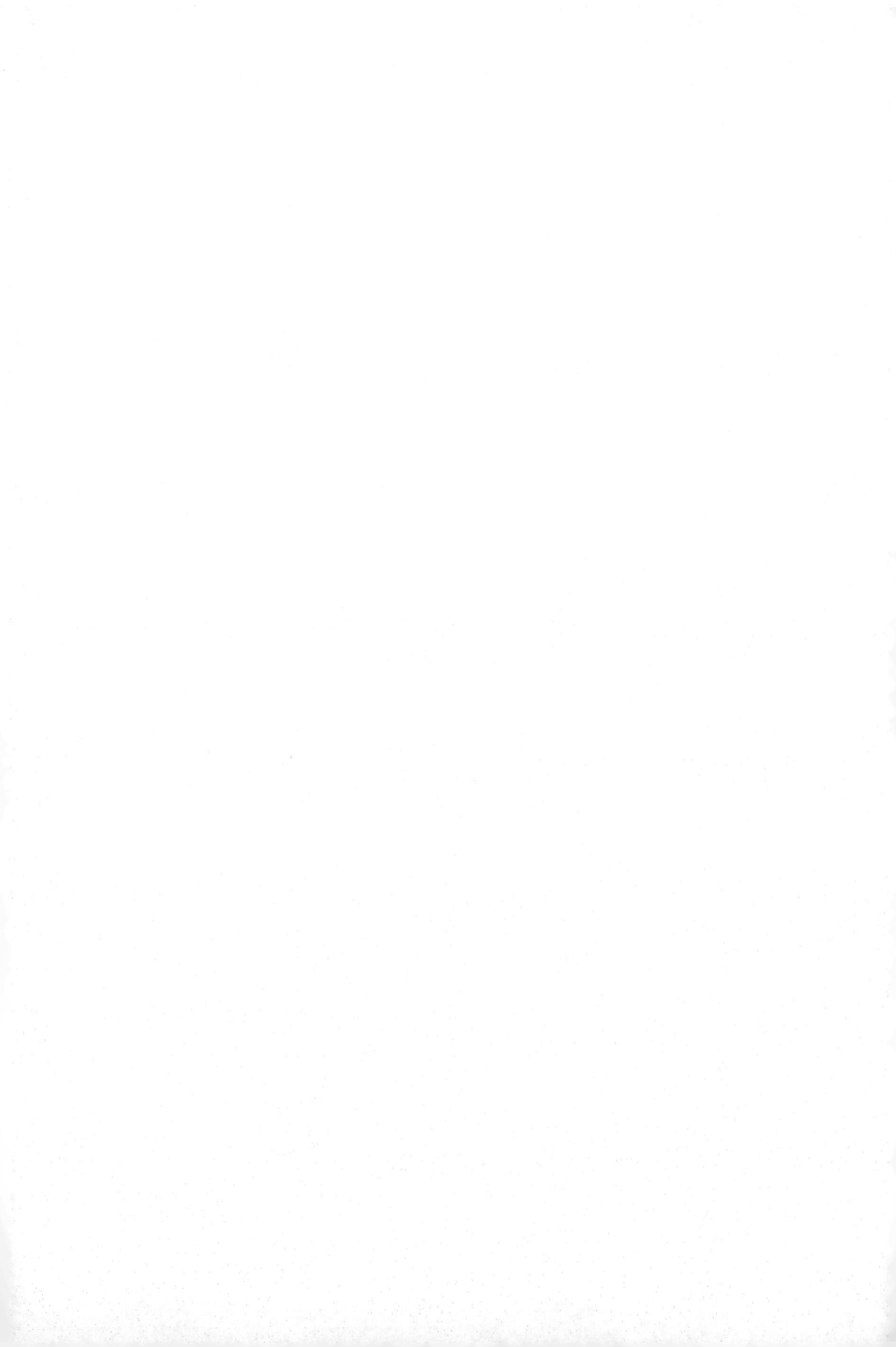